The Library
Dr Draper + partners
125 Newmarket Road
Cambridge

1919

TRANSCULTURAL MEDICINE

Dealing with patients from different cultures

Second Edition

EXTRACTS FROM REVIEWS OF THE FIRST EDITION

"Unrecognised cultural differences may, however, cause offence, resentment, or fear - unfortunate in many circumstances but especially so in medical practice, where the results may be a wrong diagnosis or treatment. Bashir Qureshi steers you cheerfully around the pitfalls."
British Medical Journal

"Sheds light on problems of communications . . . its importance extends beyond the confines of consultation between a doctor and patient."
Journal of the Royal College of General Practitioners

"This must be a book that many people have been searching for over the years."
Health Visitor

"This book is full of information, interest, and humour. It is essential reading for trainers, trainees, and established practitioners in all disciplines."
Update

". . . all health professionals dealing with the day by day situation of care in the present day 'mix' of ethnic cultures will find this book invaluable."
Journal of the Royal Society of Health

"Each page is packed with interest."
Journal of the Royal Society of Medicine

"The author should be highly commended for undertaking such painstaking research into an area of medicine which is still in its infancy."
Health and Hygiene

To all patients, colleagues, and authors
− from many ethnic groups −
who taught me a lot so as to enable me to teach others

TRANSCULTURAL MEDICINE

Dealing with patients from different cultures

Second Edition

including 35 articles published in the
British medical press 1981 – 1988

BASHIR QURESHI

FRCGP, DCH, AFOM(RCP), MFFP(RCOG), FRSH, MICGP, FRIPHH

General Practitioner and Community Health Officer, Hounslow, West London, UK
Writer, lecturer and broadcaster in Transcultural Medicine
Formerly, Member of the Council of the RCGP and its Communications, Publications and
International Committees. Editor of Faculty News. *Editor of* London Medicine.
Member of the Editorial Board of Health Trends.
Currently, Member of Council of the Royal Society of Health. Member of Council of the Society of
Public Health Medicine. Member of Council of The GP Section of the Royal Society of Medicine
and its Editorial Representative on the Journal.
Member of the BMA's Working Party on Transcultural Medicine. Deputy Medical Officer (Ethnic
Affairs) of the London Branch of the British Red Cross. An Expert Witness in Transcultural
Medicine – legal cases.

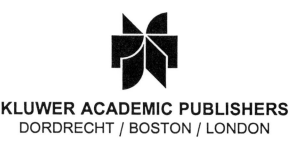

KLUWER ACADEMIC PUBLISHERS
DORDRECHT / BOSTON / LONDON

Distributors

for the United States and Canada: Kluwer Academic Publishers, PO Box 358, Accord Station, Hingham, MA 02018-0358, USA
for all other countries: Kluwer Academic Publishers Group, Distribution Center, PO Box 322, 3300 AH Dordrecht, The Netherlands

A catalogue record for this book is available from the British Library.

ISBN 0-7923-8836-4

Library of Congress Cataloging-in-Publication Data

```
Qureshi, Bashir.
    Transcultural medicine : dealing with patients from different
  cultures ; including 35 articles published in the British medical
  press, 1981-1988 / Bashir Qureshi. -- 2nd ed.
       p.    cm.
    Includes bibliographical references and index.
    ISBN 0-7923-8836-4 (casebound)
    1. Transcultural medical care.   2. Transcultural medical care-
  -Great Britain.    I. Title.
    [DNLM: 1. Delivery of Health Care.   2. Ethnic Groups.   3. Attitude
  to Health--ethnology.   4. Cultural Characteristics.    WA 300 Q9t
  1994]
  RA418.5.T73Q74    1994
  362.1'042--dc20
  DNLM/DLC
  for Library of Congress                                    93-45887
                                                                 CIP
```

Copyright

Published in the United Kingdom by Kluwer Academic Publishers,
PO Box 55, Lancaster, UK.

Kluwer Academic Publishers BV incorporates the publishing programmes of
D. Reidel, Martinus Nijhoff, Dr W. Junk and MTP Press.

Printed in Great Britain by Butler and Tanner, Frome and London.

CONTENTS

PREFACE TO THE SECOND EDITION

Culture is composed of the customs and civilization of a particular group of people. Science and religious or secular persuasions strongly influence a culture. Science is based on human observations with objectivity and reason. Religion reveals God's word; therefore, it deals with subjectivity and intuition. It is not surprising that the scientific approach is practical, analytical, rational and unemotional, whereas religious thinking is theoretical, empirical, moral and emotional. In real life, in spite of apparent contradictions, science and religion complement each other in helping a patient. Science provides material benefits and religion gives spiritual strength. Even a secular person turns to a humanist school of thought called 'rational morality'. Medicine is a science and, in fairness, it should be practised with respect to a patient's culture, religion, ethnicity, and dignity.

Ignorance of culture can lead to false diagnoses. Only by taking a full history and being sensitive to a patient's culture can a doctor make an accurate diagnosis, understand the patterns of illness in various ethnic groups, and isolate diseases which may or may not be specific to a particular ethnic group. At a plenary session of a Transcultural Medicine study day for GP trainees, a trainer told me that a 40-year old Pakistani labourer went to see his GP in Norfolk, complaining about abdominal pains, fever and debility. He was asked if he had seen blood in his stool and replied "no" because "I don't know" is seen as weakness in the Asian culture. He did not know because examining one's stool is taboo for Muslims, Hindus and Sikhs. The GP sent him to hospital for an appendix examination and the patient refused the rectal examination – another cultural taboo – and returned to his GP. He was given iron tablets as he looked pale. A blood sample was taken and he was told to return in a week. He failed to keep the appointment. Later, the GP received a hospital notification of his death from cancer of the colon.

Since the publication of the first edition, I have received much feedback in the form of reviews in numerous journals, letters from many readers, and comments from various course organizers. Dr Keith Thompson (GP and author), Sandra Barry (Practice Nurse and Midwife), and Seema Khajuria (Consultant Nutritionist) went further and wrote page-by-page commentaries. It was encouraging to note that my non-political and purely educational approach was appreciated to an extent that this book is now included in the reading lists of many clinical examinations of the Royal Colleges.

In the preparation of the second edition, many changes have been made in view of the feedback. Chapter 12 has been updated to include the disease patterns among some European ethnic groups, particularly from the European Economic Community. Chapter 14 has been re-written to describe some multicultural customs about childbirth, marriage, death, and bereavement. Some examination questions, based on real case histories, have been included so as to assist the examiners and the candidates for the undergraduate and postgraduate examination.

Finally, I reiterate my belief in Hippocrates' style of describing the first-hand observations and in writing with a sense of humour so as to promote multicultural medical understanding of all ethnic groups by a health professional of any ethnic background. The patient is the most important person in medicine and it is within the doctor's reach to provide appropriate care for each individual by learning more about his or her patient's culture. I hope you enjoy reading this book and if you have any comments, please do let me have them!

London 1994   **BASHIR QURESHI**

WHY WE MUST PRACTISE TRANSCULTURAL MEDICINE

Health professionals and GPs should concern themselves with ethnicity, religion and culture as much as with the age, sex and social class of their patients.
Transcultural medicine is the knowledge of medical and communication encounters between a doctor or health worker of one ethnic group and a patient of another. It embraces the physical, psychological and social aspects of care as well as the scientific aspects of culture, religion and ethnicity without getting involved in the politics of segregation or integration.

English general practitioners and health professionals tend to regard everyone as English, and to assume that all patients have similar needs. Would that it were as simple as that!

For economic reasons – based on supply and demand – the mass migration of working populations from the new Commonwealth countries, along with their dependent relatives (including their parents) to Britain took place during one decade – the 1960s. Broadly speaking, the workers were in their thirties and forties, and their dependent parents were in their fifties and sixties. All these will, of course, be 30 years older in the 1990s.

In fact, general practitioners and hospital consultants will see increasing numbers of people from ethnic minority groups, along with the indigenous populations. The needs of these ethnic minority citizens will differ considerably from those of the ethnic majority groups because of their different cultures, religions and ethnicity. Many doctors are scarcely aware of this trend at present; but lack of vocal demand does not mean absence of need.

TRANSCULTURAL MEDICINE

Science variables should be understood to include age, sex, social class, race, religion and culture; how can anyone call himself a scientific worker if he accepts the first three and disregards the latter variables? A multicultural approach in medicine helps in the identification, quantification and management of the problems of multi-ethnic patients, especially the elderly and women who are most likely to adhere to their own culture. Even those easterners who become westernised hardly ever change their religion and surely retain their ethnic characteristics.

"Measure what is measurable and make measurable what is not" (Galileo). My observations, made over 25 years in this less-researched area, are now open to peer audit. I do not plead for any one ethnic population or belong to any pressure group, but solely stress the need for understanding during a cross- cultural consultation in a medical setting.

WHAT'S NEW?

In this book some problems of patients from different ethnic backgrounds will be identified and quantified so as to help British health professionals and GPs – during history-taking, clinical examination, investigations and diagnosis, drug therapy and general consultation – with a clear indication of what doctors should do differently as a result of seeing how things can go wrong or be misunderstood in a particular case.

Categorisation or generalisation is the only way to measure facts and populations. Nevertheless, there remains the need to be flexible when categorising because there will be exceptions to every rule. While giving plenty of factual details, I shall be very careful when generalising about ethnic minorities as they may well differ as much between groups as they do from indigenous British people.

There is more to good quality of care than trying to save everybody's time and money. The essence of good practice must be to tailor appropriate and sensitive care to an individual situation. The art of general practice and health care goes beyond the textbooks. There is much literature on the medical model (physical, psychological and social) and, currently, increasing information is available on one-ethnic studies. This book should be considered as an addition to the existing knowledge. Properly practised, *Transcultural Medicine* highlights the interface between various cultures, asks no-one to change personal views and stays clear of discrimination, either positive or negative. It simply suggests ways of improving the quality of care by distinguishing varying needs in a cross-cultural contact, whether during a ten-minute consultation or an hour-long medical examination.

We can solve problems only if we can talk about them calmly. I should welcome communication from any readers who may have different observ-ations. Here is an opportunity for mutual learning!

London, 1989   **BASHIR QURESHI**

Part I
GENERAL ASPECTS

CHAPTER 1

AVOIDING COMMUNICATION PROBLEMS

For most GPs the practice list of today will be drawn from many ethnic backgrounds, each having a unique disease pattern related to diet, custom and physiology.

DID YOU KNOW?

- Enemas are taboo to ethnic Asians, especially women.
- Pork or beef insulin may be unacceptable to Muslims and Hindus.
- West Indians suffer from a unique form of severe hypertension.
- The retina is pink in English people but chocolate-coloured in West Indians.
- English height and weight charts do not apply to children who are ethnic Chinese, Malay, Bangladeshi, Gujarati or South Indian.
- Antibiotics, antituberculous, and antidepressant drugs show a better response but more side-effects in Afro-Asians compared with English.
- A chapati diet is exclusive to Asians, and they suffer an increased incidence of rickets because chapati flour contains phytic acid which combines with dietary calcium to make calcium phytate which is then excreted.

Some communication barriers have to be overcome before a GP consultation takes place. These can be categorised as those of language, culture, religion and social class.

Language

Even the Americans do not speak the same language as the English. How can a patient from overseas be expected to speak English in a way which should sound English to English ears?

Fortunately, most of the ethnic minority groups come from the new and old Commonwealth where English used to be the first, and is now the second, language of their country.

First published in *Pulse Reference Series*, **43**, Oct 29, 1983 (Morgan Grampian Professional Press Ltd.)

Medicine and law are still practised in English in the whole of the Commonwealth. Therefore these patients are used to having interpreters. Although the use of an interpreter, a health official or a patient's family member, may not be an ideal solution, this is a good answer to the problem in the absence of a better one.

A veterinary surgeon copes with his 'patients' and in the EEC language problems are overcome. In the same way with patience and a positive effort, language problems should not cause a deadlock in a GP consultation. As with music, sign language is universal and this can be put to good use.

Culture

Culture shock, colour shock and name shock are real entities in GP consultations, but, given time, the patient or the doctor soon gets over them.

In an Afro-Asian culture a patient expects the doctor to know the diagnosis of his problem without being questioned or examined because alternative medicine practitioners can make a good guess at their chronic conditions without this.

Moreover they would emphasise physical symptoms more than psychological ones and expect a prescription rather than mere advice because in their native culture they pay for the drugs but the consultation is free.

A few moments spent on educating the patient about the British system of supportive counselling as well as drug therapy, after having taken a detailed history and made the appropriate examination, are well worth while.

Religion

If an English GP asks an Asian or Chinese 'What is your Christian name?' he may possibly hurt their feelings because only a few such patients are Christians.

They are either Hindus, Muslims or Buddhists (atheists) and do not have the concept of Christian names; in addition, some of them have a memory of Christian missionary hospitals in their countries which in fact were associated with the British Empire, and so aggravates the feeling of hurt.

Hindus still have the caste system and a person from a lower caste may not like to tell the doctor his surname. A GP may be well-advised to ask for the first, middle and last names. Usually the first name is the given name, the middle name is the religious name and the last is the family name (surname). They would like to be addressed by their last (family) name with the appropriate title as this gives them a feeling of being treated as an adult.

Social class

Muslims, Jews and Buddhists (Chinese) do not practise a social class or caste system. Only upper-class Hindus like social class to be mentioned because they are bred to the caste system. The majority of Hindus resent the caste as well as the class system. In these circumstances, a GP would be well advised to be very careful in referring to some medical factors which are class-related.

However, lack of control of emotion and lack of vocabulary to express oneself is more common in the working class than the middle classes. Although such points help in diagnosis and treatment, they should be played down.

ETIQUETTE IN THE EXAMINATION

Greetings

The English have a 'personality profile' of vision, hearing and touch, while Africans, Asians, Chinese and East Europeans and Americans have the 'personality profile' of touch, hearing and vision.

Therefore the English will greet someone with a smile and constant eye-to-eye contact, whereas the non-English would shake hands or raise their hands and then avoid constant eye-to-eye contact.

- East Europeans (Catholics) greet with a handshake, accompanied by a warm cheek-to-cheek kiss on both sides (of course they would not do this in an English GP's surgery).
- Arabs (Muslims), Jews and Russians share the greeting with a handshake and a hug.
- Greeks: their way of greeting is to wave a clenched fist in the air and say 'Oui'. To raise an outstretched hand is a symbol of a curse – if this happens, they will cover their faces to avoid the curse.

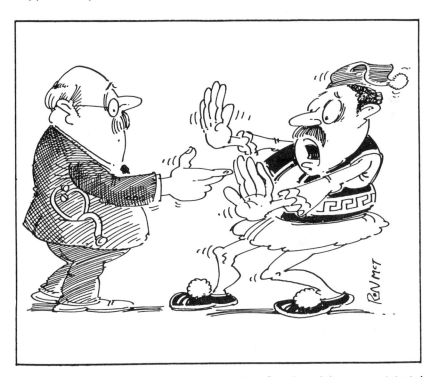

Even greetings have cultural traps . . . . to the Greek, raising an outstretched hand is a symbol of a curse

- Afro-Caribbeans (Christians) greet with a warm slapping handshake followed by a thumping of the chest, and there is a repeat of this ritual.
- Indians (Hindus) will not shake hands but will raise both hands in the position of prayer, and with a forward nodding of the head, say 'Namaskar'.
- Chinese (Buddhists) greet by clasping the hands together and bowing the head.

All of them, of course, smile after the greetings (unless they are in pain!). All this will not happen in an English GP's surgery, but if he greets patients inappropriately it may make rapport difficult. The best way to greet all patients is perhaps just to say 'Hello' with a smile and make no hand movements initially, except to indicate that the patient should take a seat.

Manners

Constant eye contact, speaking loudly, acting as a snob, holding a conversation, standing at ease with a confident smile, keeping one's hands out of one's pockets, listening and then speaking and also enjoying being quiet are all examples of English manners.

However, this is not the case in the Eastern cultures; lack of constant eye contact is a sign of respect, to be snobbish is an insult, speaking loudly is not allowed. Talking is preferred to conversation, standing to attention with a serious look, keeping one's hands in one's pockets, speaking halfway through listening and disliking being quiet are accepted norms.

Signs such as 'thumbs up', 'victory V', making a circle with the thumb and forefinger, and winking are all acceptable English gestures.

These have the opposite meanings to Easterners, who would consider 'thumbs up', encircling of thumb and forefinger and winking very rude; on the other hand, they will wave the index finger to emphasise a point, will agree on the 'victory V' sign, but may inadvertently show the reverse 'V' sign to the English GP.

If such a misunderstanding occurs, allowances should be made for cultural differences and no one should take offence.

CHAPTER 2

ETHNIC TERMINOLOGY AND OCCUPATIONS

PROBLEMS OF TERMINOLOGY AND ETHNIC GROUPS

GPs and other doctors or health care professionals will frequently have to discuss the medical problems of patients from ethnic minority groups. There is a broad range of available terminology and sometimes an inappropriate description can deeply offend a patient. The Commission for Racial Equality has considered these problems and offers the following advice. Any term that implies denigration or hatred of any ethnic group should be avoided.

- terms unacceptable: diseases in coloured people
- terms disapproved: diseases in immigrants
  reappearing diseases
  imported diseases
  alien diseases
- terms out of date   diseases in: Caucasians
  (best avoided)   Europeans
                                    English/Scottish/Welsh
- terms acceptable   diseases in: whites
  (with caution)   blacks
- *terms recommended*
  a) in Britain:
  diseases in: ethnic majority groups
                                     ethnic minority groups
                                     ethnic English, Scottish or Welsh
                                     ethnic Asian, West Indian,
                                           Chinese and so on
  b) overseas:
  diseases in: Asians, West Indians, Chinese and so on

The Commission for Racial Equality monitors the Race Relations Act. The commission was formed in 1976, replacing the Race Relations Board, and has the power to investigate a complaint about racial inequality. It takes into account not only what you say but how you say it.

First published in *Pulse Reference Series*, **43**, Oct. 29, 1983 (Morgan Grampian Professional Press Ltd.)

Occupation breakdown

The ethnic majority groups are the English, Scottish and Welsh. The popular occupations of these various ethnic groups may be of interest to the GP as well as to occupational physicians, many of whom are also GPs. The ethnic English, Scottish and Welsh are either white- or blue-collar workers; the former work in various professions such as administration, medicine, the law and legislation; the latter, for the most part, work in jobs such as in the car industry, dockyards and coalmines.

The ethnic minority groups include Irish*, Italians, Polish, Jewish, Hungarian, Afro-Caribbean, Asian, Chinese, Cypriot (Greek and Turkish) and various other small groups. The immigration pattern is occupational.

– With ethnic Irish the most popular occupations are nursing, building construction, and work in factories and pubs, and many live in Liverpool, Birmingham and Camden Town in London.
– In ethnic Asian groups the popular occupations are medicine, small businesses, restaurants and work in factories, British Rail and London Transport, and they live mostly in Southall (Punjabis), east London (Bangladeshis), Bradford (Pakistanis) and Leicester (Gujaratis).
– With ethnic West Indians the most popular occupations are nursing, working in factories, British Rail, London Transport, catering and security. In London they live in Brixton, Notting Hill Gate and Hackney. There is also a large population in Bristol.
– The ethnic Chinese mainly work in restaurants and mostly live in London, especially in the Soho area.
– Ethnic Cypriots (Greeks or Turks), Italians and Spanish work mostly in the catering industry and small businesses and live mainly in certain areas of London such as Islington.

*The Registrar General of England and Wales who uses this classification insists that the Irish are included in the ethnic minority category.

CHAPTER 3

HISTORY-TAKING AND THE EXAMINATION

History-taking

English patients are only too happy to give their life and family histories to a doctor, while Afro-Asian patients are totally unused to this routine, and view such questioning with grave suspicion.

The worst a GP can do is to ask for a passport to check the name or address. If this happens the patient may immediately walk out of his surgery. It is important to reassure the patient of the confidentiality of the information he gives, and to accept the history he gives.

Symbols may mean different things to different people. For example, to an English person, an owl is wise, a snake represents knowledge as well as healing, a cow is silly, a dog is a family pet and a black cat is a sign of good luck, whereas to an Asian patient, an owl is foolish, a snake is poisonous, a cow is sacred (Hindus), a dog is unacceptable and a black cat is a symbol of bad luck.

The word 'I' is hardly ever used by an Afro-Asian patient and 'please' and 'the' may not exist in his language (his politeness is conveyed by gesture).

The English believe strongly in the basic right of privacy, free speech, choice, the vote and the concept of queueing. These are taken very lightly in the Eastern culture.

Unlike overseas patients, the English dislike personal questions being asked in public, an aggressive approach and giving a verdict before a trial.

On the other hand, what the English like, overseas patients may dislike, such as free speech before discipline, law before religion, interest before principle, 'try before you buy' and compromise before confrontation.

Besides the above differences in concepts there are certain contradictory attitudes, for example, an English person may understate, stay cool and calm, exercise democratic discipline, believe that to err is human (mistake) and he may not give but will always forgive. Whereas a person from an Eastern culture may tend to boast, be emotional, exercise discipline democracy, may believe to err is 'demon' (sin) and he may give but will never forgive.

An English person may not like to interfere with the affairs of others; may believe in strike and counterattack and may be content to make a point indirectly, while a person from an Afro-Asian culture will choose to interfere with the affairs of others, may believe in direct action and counterpunch, and will be more forthright.

First published in *Pulse Reference Series*, **43**, Oct. 29, 1983 (Morgan Grampian Professional Press Ltd.)

An understanding of this whole series of contradictory concepts is essential if a doctor is to create a rapport with his patient. They may not have to speak the same language but should be able to understand each other.

The examination

An Eastern extended family and arranged marriage system is based on the principle of 'the less you know of others, the more you stick to one'.

Therefore a Muslim woman wears 'purdah' and a Hindu or Buddhist woman is not allowed to be alone with a man. Even a man is not used to meeting a woman alone.

Therefore, an Afro-Asian woman would prefer to be examined by a female doctor and a man would be very embarrassed if he were to be examined by a woman doctor. This may be misinterpreted by English health workers as sex discrimination but in fact nothing is further from the truth.

A rectal examination, use of enemas or suppositories and a referral to a psychiatrist are all taboo in Eastern cultures. A rectal examination is considered very insulting, while the stigma of a psychiatric referral may make a person ineligible for an arranged marriage.

If such an examination or referral is considered necessary, informative counselling should precede such an act; moreover this information must be kept in the strictest confidence, not even to be disclosed to a relative. A relative or a neighbour may hear of it and may spread gossip in the community.

In Eastern and Mediterranean cultures a husband is very possessive and may even suffer from morbid jealousy. A doctor should therefore not ignore the husband during a conversation with his wife and should never examine her without a chaperone.

In a Muslim family it is normal for the husband to speak for the whole family and for the mother to speak for the children. This may be very annoying to an English doctor. If he can understand this, he could tactfully advise the husband or the mother to be quiet during an examination, which they will happily do.

Beware of the dagger

A doctor may ask a Sikh patient to undress and may be alarmed when he sees a curved, sheathed 8-inch dagger concealed beneath his clothing! In fact, it is part of his ritual dress: all confirmed Sikhs must wear five symbols known as the five Ks – keshas (uncut hair), kangha (comb), kara (steel bangle), kachka (pair of long shorts) and kirpan (short sword).

A GP should not only control his fears, but also reassure his receptionist, who may panic.

A woman from an Eastern culture may be very shy of a vaginal examination, especially in a family planning clinic. If the receptionist or the health visitor has a word with the patient before she sees the GP, she may be prepared to co-operate.

However, if during an examination the GP faces a stumbling block, this could be overcome by deferring the examination to a later date when a relative or a religious/community leader will be available to counsel the patient. Such a counsellor will, of course, be aware of his responsibility of keeping any information confidential.

The presence of superfluous hair

This is more common in ethnic Africans, Jews, Spaniards and especially ethnic Asians. It occurs in both sexes but it is the women who seek medical advice because of its embarrassment.

It causes a great social disadvantage in an ethnic Asian adolescent girl. Her father may approach the GP as he will be very worried about its social consequences. There is a social stigma attached to a hirsute girl in that she is unlucky for the extended family and is ugly. The parents of such a girl have considerable difficulty in finding a husband for her. They have to give more Jahaiz or Dowry – a lion's share of wedding present by the bride's parents – in compensation.

In ethnic Asian children who have strictly vegetarian or vegan parents, malnutrition, especially iron deficiency anaemia, and bovine tuberculosis (glands) may be associated with transient hirsuties.

Brown colour of head lice

A head louse takes up the colour of the skin of the victim. It sucks blood from the scalp. Since the colour and composition of the blood appears to be the same in ethnic English, Asians and Africans, it is strange that the colour of the head louse is pink, brown and black respectively. Does it suck melanin pigment or is it a reflection of the victim's skin on the louse's shiny skin?

CHAPTER 4

FACTORS AFFECTING DIAGNOSIS AND HOW TO AVOID DIAGNOSTIC TRAPS

PHYSICAL DIFFERENCES

Not only are there differences in culture, food and religion between the various ethnic groups, but also there are physical differences of clinical importance.

Colour of the retina

This is directly linked to the colour of the skin, a fact not commonly known among eye specialists, let alone GPs who do not specialise in eyes.

The retina is pink in Europeans and brown in Africans. Retina colour in Asians varies according to the skin pigmentation from pink to dark brown. This could lead to the normal healthy brown of the retina of a West Indian being diagnosed as retinitis pigmentosa.

Moreover, fundoscopy to assess diabetes and hypertension may also be misinterpreted if this is not borne in mind.

However, West Indians have a genetic predisposition to a more severe form of hypertension, especially in males, and need early diagnosis as well as the appropriate treatment.

Melanisation

The factors involved in melanin pigmentation include melanocytes, steroids (adrenal cortex), melanocyte-stimulating hormone MSH (anterior pituitary), sunlight and also stress.

MSH is found as alpha and beta chains. It is secreted by the anterior pituitary, its function in humans being unknown. Possibly it is related to the metabolism of melanin pigmentation.

The chief function of melanisation is the prevention of ultraviolet photolysis of folate and other light-sensitive nutrients. Studies have shown *in vitro* that human

First published in *Pulse Reference Series*, **43**, Oct. 29, 1983 (Morgan Grampian Professional Press Ltd.)

plasma lost 30 – 50 per cent of folate in strong sunlight in one hour, and *in vivo*, ultraviolet light-treated patients show abnormally low folates.

It is reasonable to believe, given the same exposure to sunlight in people of various skin colours, that the levels of folates and other light-sensitive nutrients may be significantly different. Nevertheless this will also affect the formation of vitamin D.

Height and weight charts

Tanner's charts are based on English children from the Home Counties and these are the only charts available. These are suitable for ethnic majority groups and ethnic Afro-Caribbeans, Pakistanis and North Indians, who are all meat and wheat eaters. These are tall, light-complexioned people.

However, these charts do not apply to the Chinese, Malaysians, Sri-Lankans, Bangladeshis and South Indians, who are rice and fish eaters, and are all lightweight, short and dark-complexioned.

They also do not apply to Gujaratis from West India and East Africa, who are vegetarians, and are lightweight, short and pale-skinned.

GPs may well be aware of many problems arising when a normal, lightweight and small Gujarati, Bangladeshi or South Indian school child is found to be below the third centile on the Tanner charts. Some health visitors give great emphasis to this finding and children are subjected to specialist investigations which all prove to be normal.

Physiological lymphadenopathy

In Asian and Afro-Caribbean children, bilateral cervical and inguinal glands are normally palpable. One explanation of this is that perhaps they have small recurrent skin infections leading to this lymphadenopathy, but a more feasible explanation seems to be that the musculo-skeletal and lymphoid tissues of Afro-Asian children are more developed than in English children.

Nevertheless, a solitary cervical gland enlargement in an Asian child could be indicative of TB gland.

Mongolian spots

An Asian, Chinese or an African infant may have a large blue discoloration, especially on the buttocks, which usually disappears within one year without any treatment. This is physiological and should not be mistaken for a non-accidental injury. Simple reassurance to the mother and her mother-in-law is all that is required.

COMMON GENETIC DISORDERS AMONG ETHNIC GROUPS

Although environmental factors play a part in most conditions, there are certain conditions which are genetic.

English children

The Guthrie test is used routinely for the detection of a rise in the serum phenylalanine. Although it is a rare condition in Britain, the incidence of phenylketonuria in the United States is one in 10,000 births; the disease is transmitted by a recessive gene.

Cystic fibrosis of the pancreas, disseminated sclerosis and pernicious anaemia are said to be more common in the ethnic English than in ethnic Afro-Caribbeans and ethnic Chinese.

Ethnic Irish

Homocystinuria is an inborn error of metabolism said to be more common in the Irish and it can lead, along with other symptoms, to a characteristic shuffling or 'Charlie Chaplin' gait, and sometimes can cause mental retardation.

However, nowadays the diagnosis is likely to be made in early infancy during routine screening programmes and before clinical abnormalities have become manifest.

Ethnic Italians

Congenital dislocation of the hip is most common in Italians, especially those from Northern Italy. It is also common in Austrians. It is very rare among Afro-Caribbeans and Chinese. In Britain the incidence is around five per 1,000 live births. It is more common in females, especially those born by breech delivery.

Ethnic Jews

Tay–Sachs disease and Niemann–Pick disease are enzyme disorders more common in infants of Jewish origin, leading to eye and brain disorders. There is no treatment and death occurs within the first two or three years of life. Genetic counselling and bereavement counselling are required in such circumstances.

Ethnic Cypriots

Thalassaemia is more common in this ethnic group and is an inherited disorder of haemoglobin synthesis. Beta-thalassaemia is the commonest type and is seen in the highest incidence in peoples of Mediterranean origins, and alpha-thalassaemia is found mainly in south-east Asians. This condition invariably leads to anaemia but iron therapy is contraindicated.

It is worth remembering this possibility if faced with an anaemic patient of Afro-Asian origin. The serious type of beta-thalassaemia can occur in a child whose parents both have the thalassaemia trait. This could be avoided by genetic counselling.

Therefore, if an anaemic Cypriot child is seen the GP should not readily prescribe iron preparations in case the child is suffering from thalassaemia.

Ethnic Afro-Caribbeans

Sickle cell disease is recognised to be more significant in Afro-Caribbeans, especially those from equatorial Africa. There is a potential hazard in general anaesthesia and therefore a surgeon or dentist must be informed of this. Bloodless field surgery can be disastrous.

Haemoglobin C disease occurs almost exclusively in West Africans. However, haemoglobin D disease occurs almost exclusively in Punjabis, whereas haemoglobin E disease occurs only in Chinese. When accompanied with beta-thalassaemia, these haemoglobinopathies could become more complicated.

Glucose-6-PD deficiency is inherited as a gender-linked recessive gene and has a high incidence among Africans. In west or east Africa, as many as 20 per cent of males are affected.

Certain drugs in common use cause severe anaemia in such people, for example, antimalarials, sulphonamides, vitamin K, vitamin C and salicilates. It is interesting to note that 'Favism' (haemolytic anaemia due to broad beans) and 'phenazine' drug haemolysis (anaemia) occurs in glucose-6-PD-deficient Europeans, but not in deficient Africans.

It should be mentioned also that hernias and hydrocoeles at birth are more common in Afro-Caribbean babies.

Ethnic Asians

Haemoglobinopathy D Punjab is seen exclusively in Punjabis from Pakistan and India. It must be emphasised that these conditions are rarely seen, but are of clinical importance.

Pityriasis alba is commonly seen in ethnic Asians, usually school children, as white, scaly patches, 0.5 – 2 cm in diameter, on the face and neck. It is thought to be a variant of atopic eczema and responds well to steroids and antibiotic preparations. School teachers may mistake this for ringworm infestation, and exclude the child from school. An explanation to the school authorities will suffice.

Vitiligo is also common in ethnic Asians, and it may be a cause of considerable distress, especially when the traditional arranged marriage is affected. Lesions can be camouflaged with dihydro-acetone lotion.

Lactose intolerance is also described as being more common in Asian infants. Feeding problems among this ethnic group should be investigated with this information in mind.

As with African children, Asian children are prone to a higher incidence of the 'catarrhal child syndrome'.

Ethnic Chinese

They are most likely to have haemoglobin E disease and thalassaemia. Haemoglobin E disease is also common in people from other Far East countries. It is of special importance if inherited together with beta-thalassaemia because then the symptoms are more severe. 'Port wine stains' are apparently more common among the Chinese population.

Ethnic Vietnamese, Filipinos, Thais, Malays and Indonesians

Alpha-thalassaemia is found mainly in south-east Asia. The inheritance of this severe blood disorder from both parents is incompatible with life and such offspring are stillborn; therefore genetic counselling is essential, and in some circumstances, bereavement counselling may also be required.

CHAPTER 5

PSYCHIATRIC DISORDERS AMONG DIFFERENT ETHNIC GROUPS

Not only is the incidence of mental illness of clinical significance, but the attitude of various ethnic groups to mental illness also plays an important part.

In 1980, a survey of admissions to mental hospitals in England and Wales showed that, in comparison with the English, the admission rate among ethnic Asians was 20 per cent lower, whereas the admission rate among ethnic West Indians was 10 per cent higher. Moreover, schizophrenia was three times more common in West Indians than in English patients.

Among Asians, referral to a psychiatrist is taboo and can affect their arranged marriage prospects. Therefore, in this group more patients are treated at GPs' surgeries than are referred to psychiatrists.

Ethnic English

Men are more prone to stress and suicide, whereas women are more susceptible to depression and parasuicide. Benzene intoxication causes euphoria and occurs in industries such as rubber, plastics, paints and the byproducts of coke ovens. Women are more susceptible to this intoxication because they have more fat under the skin and benzene is fat-soluble.

In the past, rickets was known as 'the English disease', until it was replace by chronic bronchitis. Recently, however, stress has attained this distinction. Selbye coined this term in 1960.

In small doses, stress acts as a stimulant, but in excess, when it becomes strain or distress, it has pathological effects such as frustration, abnormal behaviour, anxiety, depression, alcoholism, increased susceptibility to accidents, ischaemic heart disease and psychosomatic illnesses including hay fever, asthma, eczema, peptic ulcer, spastic colon, migraine and backache.

The psychiatric hazards of various occupations should not be underestimated. Some examples, such as phobic anxiety in coal miners, or psychiatric symptoms in occupations dealing with lead, mercury, manganese, methyl bromide, carbon disulphide, vinyl chloride, methyl alcohol and nitrous oxide, as well as benzene, are worth bearing in mind, especially in those working in industrial areas.

First published in *Pulse Reference Series*, **43**, Nov. 5, 1983 (Morgan Grampian Professional Press Ltd.)

Ethnic Irish

Alcoholism is said to be most common among this group.

It is one of the five major causes of death in the UK and can result in accidents, divorce and the sack.

A social drinker can be distinguished from an alcoholic by simple observations: the former drinks small amounts at longer intervals, sipping, boasting about his intake and preferring to drink in company, whereas the latter drinks large amounts at short intervals, gulping (a glassful in one swallow!), denying that he drinks and preferring to drink alone.

Schizophrenia is also said to occur more frequently among the Irish. However, the authenticity of this point has to be further evaluated.

Ethnic Jews

Depression is said to be more common in this group than other ethnic groups in the UK. A GP practising in Golders Green is probably well aware of this.

Ethnic Poles

Paranoia is described as being more common among Poles than other ethnic groups. The term paranoia is usually applied to mental illnesses in which the predominant symptoms are persistent delusion of a persecutory or grandiose nature.

Paranoid symptoms may occur in a variety of conditions and where paranoid features include delusions, the term 'paranoid psychosis' is applicable. Paranoid states are not disease entities in themselves but may occur in many mental illnesses including 'paranoid reaction' and 'paranoid personality'.

'Paranoid reaction': it is possible for someone to develop a paranoid state as a reaction to some stress. In such a case there is often a constitutional predisposition to react in this way, but when delusions develop the condition may be indistinguishable from paranoid schizophrenia. Some of these cases were often labelled 'paranoia' in the past.

'Paranoid personality': this is a personality disorder which occasionally spills over into a paranoid reaction following psychological or environmental stress. There are two type of paranoid personality:

– Sensitive and suspicious

– Individuals who cling to some belief or cause tenaciously, often having 'overvalued ideas' which do not amount to delusions. These people are frequently 'anti-this' or 'anti-that' and go through life with a very large chip on their shoulders.

Ethnic Hungarians

Like other East Europeans, Hungarians have a greater incidence of suicide than other ethnic groups. Hungary is the richest country in the Communist bloc; suicide rates are highest among the upper class.

Another example is that of Sweden, which is one of the richest countries in the world and has the highest incidence of suicide. Suicide in Europeans is commoner in the spring and is the fifth commonest cause of death in Britain among young people.

Ninety per cent of suicides have been suffering from a mental disorder, psychotic depression and alcoholism and the majority have been in touch with their family doctor or with a hospital outpatients' clinic in the preceding month.

Elderly males living in social isolation are at greater risk. Suicide rates tend to be higher in areas of social disorganisation or in the bedsitter/lodging house areas of large cities (e.g. Earls Court).

Although there is a higher rate among all immigrants, it seems that it is highest in Hungarians and other East Europeans.

Ethnic Cypriots, Greeks, Turks and Italians

All have a higher incidence of morbid jealousy – the 'Othello' syndrome – than other groups. It is more common in men.

A man possessed with such jealousy may show aggressive behaviour because of his conviction – delusional or otherwise – that his wife is unfaithful.

As a typical case, a man in his 40s, after about six years of marriage, may suffer with morbidly jealous delusions and he may go on for another four years before he acts in an aggressive way. Fortunately most patients suffer mildly and simple reassurance is sufficient, but in severe cases, the only preventive measure is separation or divorce.

It is advisable for an English doctor, when speaking to a woman of one of these ethnic groups, not to ignore her male partner. And it is wiser not to be alone with her. A GP who examines such a woman without a chaperone may be taking a great risk.

Ethnic Afro-Caribbeans

Acute psychotic episodes, schizophrenia and behavioural problems among adolescents are said to be most common in this ethnic group.

Acute psychotic episodes are encountered in Afro-Caribbeans; an adolescent may go berserk. This condition presents as schizophrenia, but responds to the treatment of depression. It lasts for six weeks but seldom recurs.

In immigrant communities such as West Indians their previous culture has a strong effect on their illnesses which tend to be coloured by their previous background and superstitions. In many developing countries, for example, a belief in the prevalence of witches, demons, ghosts and other supernatural agencies is widespread.

Moreover the concept of spirit-possession is taken for granted as a relatively common experience. Not surprisingly, as with ethnic Asians or ethnic Chinese, an Afro-Caribbean woman may come to see the GP and complain that her mother-in-law or a relative or neighbour has cast a spell on her, which is the root of all her ills.

If an English doctor does not listen to her and give supportive counselling, it likely that she may turn to alternative medicine.

Recent studies have shown that schizophrenia is three times more common among West Indians than the ethnic English. This illness has genetic as well as environmental aetiology.

Adolescent identity crises, delinquency, truancy and agressive behaviour among West Indian adolescents is said to be more common. A GP who can be tolerant and sympathetic towards these adolescents can do a lot to shape their behaviour.

Ethnic Asians

Conversion hysteria is most common in Asian women, especially in girls who feel the stress of a two-culture conflict – an Asian discipline at home and English freedom with her peers at school or work.

The *Kama Sutra* is a popular book among Asians but impotence is a common problem. Premarital sex is a cultural taboo, whereas sex within marriage is considered to be a duty.

The anxiety and stress of the responsibility of an extended family system may cause loss of libido in men. They may ask the GP for an aphrodisiac before turning to alternative medicine. All that is required is supportive counselling.

In an arranged marriage system it is paramount that the bride is a virgin. The extended family system exercises a severe control over sexual behaviour, in some cases to such an extent that a woman becomes frigid and needs psychological treatment after marriage.

The mentally handicapped are considered to be 'saints' in an Asian community. They are well looked after by the family in return for their blessings and the good luck they are supposed to bestow.

Ethnic Sri-Lankans

Recent studies have revealed that schizo-affective disorders are more common in the women than men of this group.

Some diseases are said to be less common in ethnic Asians. Examples are the Oedipus complex, abnormal reactions to bereavement, suicide, and anxiety neuroses. These are thought to be less common because in times of stress their religious beliefs and the extended family system provide individual psychotherapy and group therapy.

Male homosexuality and lesbianism are forbidden in Asian culture. The extended family system helps prevents marital breakdown and divorce by relieving the financial pressure on the newly-married couple. It is customary after marriage for the bridegroom to stay with his own parents until he is financially stable, but for the bride to spend half the time with her own parents and the rest with her in-laws.

It is only when they buy or rent their own house that they are allowed to live together and the 'holidays' at parental homes become optional. It follows therefore that marital pathology is less common in this group.

Chinese, Vietnamese, Filipinos, Thais, Malays and Indonesians

'Unusual forms of mental illness' are said to occur. These can be produced by various cultural effects especially a belief in witches, demons and black magic, for example:

– Malays;
  Koro (similar to castration fear)
  Latah (compulsive movements)

– Chinese and Indonesians;
  Voodoo (magical death due to intense fear, e.g. when a person thinks he has been bewitched) – all groups.

Although depression, schizophrenia and abnormal emotional reactions are present in all groups, their incidence varies greatly among the different ethnic groups. In addition, certain ethnic groups have unusual forms of psychological illnesses due to their beliefs and customs.

CHAPTER 6

DIET-RELATED DISEASES

An awareness of ethnic diets and the possibility of related disease patterns can be of great value in investigation and treatment of ethnic patients.

You are what you eat; a balanced diet is essential for health. Variety is the spice of life and, in England, various ethnic diets have become increasingly popular. However, in spite of their good nutritional value, they seem to bring hazards of varying degrees.

Medical emergencies

There are three ethnic foods which can cause medical emergencies: karela – a vegetable; ackee – a fruit, and vetsin – an additive.

Karela is a popular choice of vegetarian Hindus (Indians) and is cooked in a curry. This vegetable has a marked hypoglycaemic effect; it has been used in place of insulin by Hakims in old Indian therapies.

It can potentiate the action of oral hypolgycaemics and cause prolonged hypoglycaemia, resulting in faintness or coma. In the differential diagnosis of fainting or coma, this possibility should be included. In mild cases a patient may come to the surgery complaining of feeling weak. This should be differentiated from the symptoms of anaemia or depression before embarking on investigations or treatment.

Ackee is a fruit eaten as a native delicacy in Jamaica. If picked unripe, from plants, and uncooked, it is so poisonous it can kill. Therefore, children are not allowed near its forbidden plants. However, when it is ripe and cooked well, it is quite delicious.

Three-quarters of the West Indians in the UK are from Jamaica. Poisoning with this food should be borne in mind when seeing an ethnic Jamaican patient with symptoms of food poisoning.

Vetsin is a sauce provided in Chinese restaurants. It contains monosodium glutamate and some people are allergic to it. This allergy can take the form of such symptoms as a thumping headache lasting for half an hour. This condition is known as the 'Chinese restaurant syndrome'.

Although these are rare emergencies, in multi-ethnic areas such information can be lifesaving. No-one, but no-one, can overestimate the role of a GP interested in ethnic health issues.

First published in *Pulse Reference Series*, **43**, Nov. 5, 1983 (Morgan Grampian Professional Press Ltd.)

Hazards of popular ethnic diets

Four ethnic diets are worth mentioning: English, African, Indian and Chinese. It is their carbohydrate content when taken in excess which leads to chronic diseases. These are potatoes (English), cassava (African), chapati (Indian) and rice (Chinese).

Potatoes: Current scientific evidence suggests that an excess of potatoes is as harmful as bread or sugar; potato starch is converted into glucose, surplus glucose is converted into fat and the excess of fat is associated with the risk of coronary heart disease, which is the biggest killer disease in the UK, escpecially in middle-aged European men, who are most needed by their families.

Multi-ethnic observations revealed that bread and sugar are consumed by all ethnic groups, but the English eat more potato chips than ethnic Asians, Africans or Chinese in this country.

The daily requirement of carbohydrates is about 375 g. The use of potatoes within its limit is justified, but exceeding this limit is a serious health hazard and must be discouraged.

Cassava (Mohogo): This is mainly consumed by Afro-Caribbeans. It contains very small amounts of thiocyanates, and when eaten over a long period can cause pancreatic diabetes.

Chapati: Eaten as a staple diet exclusively by ethnic Asians as their main bread in unlimited amounts. It contains phytic acid which combines with calcium in the diet to make calcium phytate and this cannot be absorbed by the gut and is therefore excreted.

This factor, in addition to a lack of vitamin D and calcium supplements in the diet, can lead to three things: foetal rickets, childhood rickets (one to four years of age – this is the time when an Asian infant is introduced to chapatis), and osteomalacia in adults.

In women, osteomalacia can lead to a small pelvis, therefore necessitating a caesarian section birth, whereas in the elderly it can lead to osteoporosis. It is not enough to give vitamin D but it is essential to supplement the calcium in the diet to get over this problem.

Rice: The main carbohydrate of Chinese food, for reasons yet to be discovered, may cause post-bulbar duodenal ulcers.

Perhaps it would be wise to have a portion of each of these ethnic foods rather than stick to only one.

Appraisal of ethnic diets

Common ethnic diets are English, Italian, Greek, vegetarian, vegan, Indian and Chinese.

English food: Generally provides a balanced diet and is light enough to keep a person awake at work in the afternoons, but it is low in fibre which can lead to constipation and all its attendant problems.

Italian food: Contains pasta which is described as being an ideal food for a marathon runner because of its consistent calorie supply. However, the diet contains excess fat which leads to obesity and cardiac problems.

Greek food: Economical and tasty, but it contains excessive amounts of olive oil which can cause loose motions, leading to reduced absorption of essential nutrients and prescribed drugs.

Vegetarian and Chinese food: Both have a high fibre content which avoids constipation but results in low weight gain, leading to physiological light weight and short stature.

Vegan food: Contains no eggs, cheese or milk and obviously very low in cholesterol, but without the binding ingredients the stools are extremely liquid with again the problems of reduced absorption of essential nutrients and recommended drugs. This can even interfere with growth patterns.

Indian food: Is economical, filling and tasty but has highly-spiced ingredients and large quantities of herbs which can cause the curry smell, not only from the mouth, but also through the breath and the skin. This could be objectionable to anyone who has not eaten the same food.

All ethnic diets contribute to the quality of life and provide a sensory change. Nevertheless, there are shortcomings which, if one is aware of them, can be dealt with.

Dietary habits

These vary in different ethnic groups. For example, for eating rice, the English will use a fork, Afro-Asians will use a spoon and the Chinese prefer chop-sticks.

Whereas the English use a knife and fork, Afro-Asians may use clean hands for eating. According to religious and cultural customs they wash their hands before eating, and after eating they not only wash their hands again but also rinse their mouths, thereby cleaning the teeth.

It is said that this habit is the reason for their strong teeth. No wonder they can tear the meat with their teeth and do not need cutlery − which, in a large family, they sometimes cannot afford anyway.

Some children who do not wash their hands, or who have long nails which they have not cleaned, could get tummy upsets.

Ethnic Chinese, Malaysians and Indonesians all use chop-sticks. In this way they can take in only small amounts of food at one time, allowing more time for the food to mix with saliva. They reach satiety with smaller amounts of food with this method.

A GP should not take it for granted that all his ethnic patients will be eating by one method. He may be approached by the home help or catering in GP hospitals for advice. It is important for a patient to use his ethnic method of eating when he is ill, rather than be forced to eat with a knife and fork.

Ethnic nutritional problems in schools

Religious taboos: a GP may be contacted by a head teacher for advice on the provision of meals and problems of ethnic diets. It is an advantage to know some religious taboos, for example, Muslims and Jews do not eat pork, Hindus are forbidden to eat beef, vegetarians do not eat meat, vegans do not even have eggs or cheese, Jehovah's Witnesses refuse to eat black pudding. Such points can cause problems in school children, especially when on special diets for diabetes or obesity.

Cultural taboos: in Afro-Asian culture, milk, orange juice, lemonade and Ribena are considered drinks which aggravate colds and coughs. Therefore the parents will write a note to the teacher forbidding them to supply these to their children at school. A teacher, unaware of this custom, may be annoyed and may ring the GP for advice. A simple explanation to both parties is all that is needed.

Vegetarian children are prone to iron deficiency anaemia and children eating curry may develop halitosis and require vigorous oral hygiene.

Muslims observe fasting (Ramadan), Christians and Hindus observe Lent. Hindus and Sikhs may hesitate to eat with Muslims. Lightning hunger strikes are a manner of protest by Asian children.

An understanding and appropriate management of these situations wherever they arise can resolve many conflicts. At present, health visitors, school nurses and head teachers when faced with such situations contact the GP for advice.

Ethnic groups... diets and disease

We are aware that certain illnesses such as anaemia, allergy, cancer, heart disease, migraine and peptic ulcer are related to diet. However, certain ethnic groups consume more of certain foods. A food may be related to a disease which could therefore be more prevalent in a particular population.

Ethnic English: Consume more tea, milk, eggs, animal fats, chicken, sugar, chocolate and potatoes than other ethnic groups. Recent studies suggest that tea is related to constipation; milk and eggs contain substances which could cause allergies such as eczema in some cases; a high content of animal fat in the diet could lead to ischaemic heart disease, cancer of the colon and loose motions (interfering with the absorption of food and drugs); chicken not properly thawed from a frozen state could lead to food poisoning; sugar and chocolate can cause dental caries; potatoes, especially fried chips, can lead to obesity.

Ethnic Irish: Drink more alcohol than other ethnic groups. Alcohol can cause cirrhosis of the liver and malnutritional anaemia, and along with the latter, increased susceptibility to infections, especially tuberculosis.

Ethnic East Europeans: Drink more coffee than other ethnic groups. It has been suggested that excessive coffee-drinking could be related to cancer of the pancreas.

Ethnic Afro-Caribbeans: Take more salt in their diets. Salt is related to hypertension and ethnic Afro-Caribbeans have a genetic predisposition to this, which is more severe in males.

Ethnic Asians: Use a lot of onion, garlic and chillies in curries. Although onion and garlic are said to lower blood pressure, they can cause the lingering smell of curry on the breath. Chillies, red or green, could cause flatulent dyspepsia or intestinal hurry. In treating these conditions, antacids are more effective than anti-diarrhoeals.

Ethnic Japanese: Are used to having raw fish in their diet, and this is described as causing peptic ulcer and cancer of the stomach. It should be remembered that some Japanese may continue to eat their usual diet while on business trips to the UK.

An awareness of ethnic diets and the possibility of diet-related disease patterns could be of great value in the investigation and treatment of illness in ethnic patients.

CHAPTER 7

AVOIDING DIAGNOSTIC TRAPS RELATED TO CUSTOMS

People have immigrated from all the five continents at various times in British history, just as the British have emigrated to all parts of the world. Native cultural heritages and customs are the most valuable possessions of all ethnic groups.

Problems can occur when a doctor of one culture is dealing with a patient of another culture. To describe all the customs of all cultures represented in the UK is not possible in this series.

Nevertheless, some examples of cultural customs giving rise to health hazards can be described to help avoid diagnostic traps.

These are categorised under the headings of personal, extended family and community.

PERSONAL

A culture may expect its individuals to behave in a prescribed fashion and GPs may see patients from different cultures who indulge in some of the following habits.

Betel chewing

This is an after-dinner delicacy practised by adult Asians and Malaysians. According to the *Encyclopaedia Britannica*, one tenth of the world's population practises this habit.

A betel leaf is used as a wrapper and the contents include betel nut, tobacco, limestone paste, catechu, cardomum, rose hips, turmeric root and silver foil. It is interesting to note the functions of these ingredients.

Betel leaf, cardomum and rose hips are mainly carminatives, a source of vitamin C, and provide a pleasant odour. They also increase the salivary secretions. For astringent action betal nut and catechu are included. Limestone paste is a rich source of calcium which prevents osteomalacia, foetal rickets and calcium deficiency in the elderly.

First published in *Pulse Reference Series*, **43**, Nov. 5, 1983 (Morgan Grampian Pprofessional Press Ltd.)

These three diseases, with childhood rickets, are not only related to vitamin D deficiency but also to the 'chapati diet' – an exclusive diet of Asians, as described in Chapter 6.

To protect against damage to the buccal mucosa by limestone paste, catechu is added, which itself is a rich source of iron, thereby preventing iron deficiency anaemia. Tobacco is an important ingredient; nicotine is a stimulant in small doses. Turmeric root is used for colouring.

Lastly, silver foil, and sometimes gold foil – a thin film is used to wrap the betel leaf with its contents. Not only is this of aesthetic value, but also it is considered to be aphrodisiac. A special receptacle is used for spitting out the remains. Some people use this after-dinner delicacy to entertain guests. Therefore spitting in public is an acceptable practice for that culture as long as the appropriate receptacle is provided.

As long as betel chewing is kept in proportion, it serves a healthy purpose, but when it exceeds the limit, there are three health hazards.

First, the astringents, especially the betel nut, are described as predisposing to gallstones, renal stones and stones in the bladder. When treating such patients, a GP should advise stopping betel chewing. The medical treatment of gallstones and other stones for that matter may be unsuccessful if a patient continues to chew betel in unlimited amounts.

Second, limestone paste is a strong irritant to the buccal mucosa. A person who keeps on chewing betel as a nervous habit is likely to retain its contents for a long time in his mouth, between the gums and the cheek. The buccal mucosa may be eroded by limestone paste and develop into a chronic ulcer. If this ulcer is not treated adequately it may develop carcinogenic changes. In the betel-chewing population, cancer of the cheek is common. The GP should bear this clinical point in mind.

Third, an Asian patient may emphatically deny smoking; Sikhs do not smoke, as a religious taboo. However betel chewing is practised by people from all Asian cultures. An English GP should always bear this source of tobacco consumption in mind when investigating a patient with cancer or other problems usually associated with tobacco.

Hooka smoking

English GPs may remember the hooka-smoking caterpillar in *Alice's Adventures in Wonderland*. This is a popular social custom among many Asians, especially the men.

The hooka is a smoking apparatus consisting of a flask filled with water with two tubes attached. One tube is topped by a funnel which contains lighted coals, under which there is a metal lid above a layer of tobacco paste, and its lower end is under the water.

One end of the second tube is above the water; the other end is fitted with a mouthpiece like that of a pipe. Tobacco vapour filtered through the water is inhaled through this mouthpiece. It is useful to remember this source of smoking when taking a patient's history, especially with an elderly person. There are many designs of the hooka.

'Surma' eye make-up

This is a lead powder, usually imported from India, used as an eye-liner for infants and Asian women. Through contact with the fingers when being applied, or when a child sucks its thumb, it can be ingested, causing varying degrees of lead toxicity.

A GP should advise replacing the 'Surma' with 'Kajal' which is made of ash collected from a 'Diva' – an Asian oil lamp commonly used at the time of the Divali festival. Kajal is sold commercially and is safe and inexpensive, and provides a satisfactory substitute eye make-up.

Antimony teeka

This is a red spot worn on the forehead of Hindu women. A married Hindu woman will wear, in addition, 'Sandoor' – antimony powder in the parting line of her hair, as long as her husband is alive. Occasionally, metal-induced allergic dermatitis can occur.

Sarsoon oil

In the Asian sub-continent, prolonged exposure to sunshine causes dryness of the skin. To counteract this, it is customary to apply sarsoon oil all over the body. It is cheap, readily available and very effective. However, it has a specific smell. As with smokers or curry eaters, as long as everybody uses it, nobody notices it!

However, this smell may not be acceptable to English people. A GP can advise such a patient to substitute this imported oil with suitable moisturising lotions. This problem can also occur in mixed schools and a GP attached to such a school can counsel the teachers as well as the parents.

Toilet habits

An Asian, African or Chinese patient may prefer to have a shower rather than a bath because they are brought up not to sit in used bath water. The bath is a Western custom, though an English person is happy to use a shower.

Hospital doctors and nurses, as well as GPs, should not try to persuade an ethnic minority patient to use a bath in preference to a shower.

The English prefer a lavatory with a high seat, and use toilet paper, though they are now acquiring the Continental habit of using a bidet for cleansing. Ethnic minority patients, especially Asians, are accustomed to using low-seat lavatories, followed by a wash with plenty of water instead of paper. It is said that the incidence of haemorrhoids is less among Asians due to this reason, apart, perhaps, from those who have adopted Western ways.

In factories where Asians work and the management do not consider their needs as different from those of the English, a special problem occurs. Either an Asian/Chinese employee will make excuses to go home in order to use his Asian-style lavatory or he will take an empty container such as a milk bottle which he fills with water in order to wash.

This innocent improvisation causes great surprise and confusion to English co-workers. An occupational physician in this situation could mediate to counsel an employer to provide both Western and Eastern style lavatories.

Western men prefer to stand to urinate while Eastern men prefer to sit. Therefore it is not unusual to see a queue of Asian men waiting to use the only closet, while a row of urinals stands empty.

These situations may arise in places of work, hospitals and newly-built GP health centres.

Non-words

'Please' and 'the' are non-words in Eastern languages. However, 'please' is expressed by gestures. Allowances should be made for this apparent lack of courtesy.

Personal questions

It is not uncommon for a GP to be asked very personal questions by an Asian patient, such as his salary, private life, value of his premises and property, and date of retirement. Some receptionists who work with overseas-trained GP locums, when faced with these questions, recommend to their principals never to employ that locum again. If only they knew!

In fact people from Eastern cultures worship authority, including the doctor, and this is an innocent manner of getting to know a person, because they prefer to talk about concrete facts rather than abstract matters. This is purely a cultural difference and is in no way intended to cause distress or embarrassment.

A GP should be forthcoming in advising such a patient or overseas-trained doctor not to ask these personal questions, advice which he will readily take.

Cosmetic problems

Ear piercing: This is common in all ethnic groups but an Asian may have each ear pierced in as many as five or six places to wear expensive golden earrings.

Nose piercing: This is not practised in Western or Chinese cultures, but in England barbers provide the service for nose-piercing as with ear-piercing, and charge approximately £5. It is also carried out in high-class jewellery shops. Nose piercing is popular among Asians and Afro-Caribbeans, and of course recently among punks.

Ceremonial scars: These are carried out among Africans from certain tribes. A patient will be very offended if a GP denigrates these scars.

Female circumcision: This controversial practice is dying out. It has been carried out by certain African tribes. In my view, the move to have this practice banned by legislation appears to be an over-reaction.

Hair plaiting: This is very popular among Afro-Caribbeans, especially children and women. Sometimes alopecia may result from this practice. At the time of examination, the patient's hair may not be plaited, but this point should be queried.

Binding of feet: This is another example of a custom that has died out. The Chinese used to bind the feet of female children because they believed that small feet were an indication of beauty and aristocracy.

Glue sniffing: Although there is said to be a higher incidence of glue sniffing among English and Scottish children, this habit is now spreading to other groups.

Henna dyeing: An English GP may be very surprised to see an Asian woman with red hair. In fact some of them are very conscious of grey hair and it is the custom to dye such hair red. Similarly, he may see an Eastern man dyeing his beard red for the same reason and should be able to distinguish between true redheads and pseudo-redheads.

It is also customary for Asian women and girls to dye their hands, feet and nails with henna, thereby making physical examination a little bit more complicated. Western women, and nowadays even Western men, are more fond of dyeing their hair than Afro-Caribbeans and Chinese.

Extended family roles

In Western culture, the concept of the nuclear family is more popular; a man and a woman and two children. In Eastern and Afro-Caribbean cultures, the extended family concept persists. The man is the breadwinner and taxpayer.

The wife is in charge of all home affairs. All the relatives are interdependent socially, culturally and financially. In the West, everone looks after themselves and as a result an improved society prevails. In the East, everyone looks after someone else and their pay-off is a closeknit family. There are advantages and disadvantages in both systems.

In an English family, the husband and wife both have equal say – some may argue the extent of this. In Asian/Chinese families, the father dominates and a strict discipline is enforced in the house. Afro-Caribbean families are female-dominated just as the Jewish and Americans are said to be.

Afro-Caribbean teenagers who are educated in England, especially the males, resist this maternal domination. They collude with the father to form an 'opposition'. Of course, this may not be the whole story.

Health authorities who can understand these socio-psychological patterns will be more successful in shaping the behaviour of these youngsters who want equality in their own homes.

Birth: In Eastern cultures, when a child is born the relatives play a supportive role. The mother is nursed at home for about 40 days by her female relatives, especially her female in-laws.

Her grandmother plays the role of a health visitor, night-nurse, caretaker, baby minder and family counsellor. A GP visiting an ethnic minority patient should always respect the grannie.

Marriage: Marriage means different things to different people. Some people believe a man is not complete until he is married and then he is finished. Of course the same can also be said of a woman. To an English person, marriage is the result of freedom of choice. This right is valued dearly and follows the principle of 'try before you buy'.

In Eastern cultures this is not the case. The right of society overtakes the right of the individual. Marriages are arranged after thoughtful consultations between the two families concerned. They believe that 'the less you know of others, the more you stick to one'. Therefore they act upon the practice of buying and then trying.

Both systems have merits and demerits. Both aim for a stable marriage and family life. However, it may not be far from the truth to say that 'relatives you get and friends you choose'.

In the Western culture both partners are usually working, therefore financial contributions to the household are shared.

In Eastern cultures, only the man is working and therefore to supplement his earnings it is customary for a bride to come to the marriage with a dowry – the amount varies according to the means of the bride's relatives.

Bereavement: In the West, bereavement counselling is carried out by the GP or some relatives. The three stages of bereavement are now well recognised. In Eastern cultures, bereavement counselling is conducted by members of the extended family.

The funeral is followed by burial if they are Muslims and cremation if they are Hindus, and takes place on the day of death. All the relatives and friends try to attend the funeral. For the next three days, some relatives and friends gather every morning to talk about the deceased and other deceased persons, at the house of the deceased.

Meals for all those attending are provided by the immediate family. This becomes a sort of group therapy. On the third day, a larger get-together of relatives and friends takes place as an expression of sympathy to the bereaved.

After that, every morning for a period of 10 days, the women, and men who are not at work, get together to console the bereaved and talk again about their own relatives who have died. On the 10th day the bereavement is declared closed. Thereafter, anniversaries of the day of death are celebrated, contrary to Western customs.

In the East, birthdays are not celebrated, even in childhood. It is relevant to note here that in the West birthdays are celebrated, but the anniversaries of death are not, whereas in the East the opposite is the case. However, there are some Westernised Eastern people who would celebrate both.

The GP who is aware of these cultural differences can anticipate when he should contact the bereaved, and what importance to give to birthdays or death anniversaries, and when to expect the need for bereavement counselling. Community matters are described later on.

CHAPTER 8

DISEASES RELATED TO VISITS TO COUNTRY OF ORIGIN

Many members of ethnic minority groups take their long holidays in their countries of origin in Asia, Africa, the West Indies, China and south-east Asia. Many English people work in Third World countries as missionaries, for example, and take long holidays in England.

Moreover many English people go abroad to these countries on holiday. Medical problems can occur in all these groups and can present to the British GP.

It is not my intention to describe the whole range of tropical diseases in this book and it is relevant to confine discussion to the problems faced in the UK.

Nevertheless, a short list of rare diseases which occur in Third World countries but are hardly ever seen by the British GP include:

Burkitt's lymphoma	Plague
Cholera	Rabies
Fly-spread food poisoning	Tropical ulcers
Kala Azar	Trypanosomiasis
Kwashiorkor	Yaws
Kangri cancer	Yellow fever
Lassa fever	Scorpion and snake bites
Marasmus	

Rare diseases must be born in mind.

An overall view of common diseases which a British holiday-maker returning from abroad, or travellers arriving from abroad may present with, is described here.

Acute abdomen

A GP may be called out at night to a patient in a nearby hotel or a neighbourhood where various ethnic groups live. The patient may have an acute

First published in *Pulse Reference Series*, **43**, Nov. 12, 1983 (Morgan Grampian Professional Press Ltd.)

abdomen. In addition to the differential diagnoses applicable to an English patient, one should consider the following possibilities.

Common:
- Abdominal tuberculosis
- Amoebic dysentery, peritonitis as well as caecal or duodenal chronic amoebiasis
- Helminthiasis
- Schistosomiasis
- Sickle cell disease – abdominal crisis
- Typhoid fever – perforation

Rare:
- Actinomycosis of ileo-caecal region
- Burkitt's lymphoma
- Gallstones
- Hydatid cysts
- Thalassaemia major in infants
- Volvulus – sigmoid or caecum

Surgical conditions

Some surgical conditions are more common in ethnic minority groups who reside in Britain and holiday in their country of origin, and travellers who reside in those countries and holiday in Britain. Sometimes an English person working or holidaying abroad may also present with these conditions:

Hydrocoele: this condition is more common in West Indians and on transillumination it has been observed that there is more transmission of light than in other ethnic groups. As one proceeds from temperate climates towards the Equator, the incidence of vaginal hydrocoele increases. Rare conditions such as filariasis should be borne in mind and these account for 80 percent of hydrocoeles in some tropical countries.

Post-bulbar duodenal ulcer: recent radiological investigations suggest that this condition is more common among the rice-eating populations which include Bangladeshis, Japanese, Chinese, Malaysians, South Indians and West Indians.

Hernias: all hernias are more common in ethnic West Indians and it is common to see umbilical hernias in West Indian infants. Para-umbilical hernia is the one most likely to become strangulated. Perhaps one should actively look for this in such ethnic patients.

Less common conditions among ethnic minorities

- Appendicitis
- Atherosclerosis
- Carcinoma   – basal cell
                             – breast
                             – colon
                             – cervix

- Dental diseases
- Diverticular disease
- Haemorrhoids
- Peptic ulcer (gastric)
- Phimosis and para-phimosis
- Varicose veins

Medical conditions

There are certain common conditions that one should keep in mind.

Turberculosis: pulmonary and non-pulmonary tuberculosis are prevalent in the Third World and in India and Pakistan there is high mortality and morbidity due to this. The reason for this is multi-factorial. The factors include over-population, poverty, inadequate preventive and therapeutic measures, impure oral medications (necessitating the use of injections), low body resistance and high disease exposure.

Ethnic Asians residing in the UK have low resistance to tuberculosis and in spite of having had BCG inoculations, they may not have sufficient resistance to combat the high exposure to *Myobacterium tuberculosis* which they may face when visiting some rural parts of India and Pakistan.

In India there is an additional problem. The cow is sacred and is a family's most beloved possession. Usually, cows are inoculated against tuberculosis but the milk is not pasteurised. At times, some cows escape this rigorous inoculation procedure. It is the custom for guests to have the pleasure of drinking cow's milk straight from the udder. This is considered a treat. These factors could lead to bovine tuberculosis.

It is not uncommon for a British GP to see an ethnic Asian patient with non-pulmonary tuberculosis, especially that of neck glands, intestines, kidney, spine and tuberculous meningitis. It is not sufficient to heave a sigh of relief when the chest X-ray is normal.

Malaria: recently, medical journals have described many cases of malaria in people returning from holidays abroad. Rare cases include an infant receiving an exchange transfusion from a donor who suffered from malaria. Diagnostic pitfalls are such that cerebral malaria could be mistaken for sub-arachnoid haemorrhage.

Food-poisoning: many Hindus visit the River Ganges. Many Muslims go on pilgrimages to Mecca. Many English people go on holiday to tropical countries. Although every effort is made by the health authorities to maintain a good standard of hygiene for travellers, this may sometimes be inadequate. Some pilgrims may bring back holy water from shrines, but during travel, refrigeration facilities may not be up to standard. Some patients returning from these trips may complain of food poisoning with *S. typhimurium.*

Typhoid fever: for the same reasons, some patients may contract typhoid fever or become carriers. Chloramphenicol is the empirical treatment for this condition.

Amoebic dysentery: in some places where water purification is not adequate, not only bacillary dysentery but also amoebic dysentery may prevail, and should not be mistaken for ulcerative colitis, and full investigations should be carried out.

Tropical ulcers: due to the intense heat, some ethnic minority patients who reside in the UK and have low acclimatisation to heat may develop tropical ulcers when holidaying in tropical countries. These are multiple and may leave ugly scars which take a long time to disappear. Confusion may result if school teachers think these scars represent an unknown tropical disease. A school doctor or GP can reassure them.

CHAPTER 9

THERAPY AND MULTI-ETHNIC GROUPS: FACTORS AFFECTING TREATMENT

RELIGIOUS TABOOS

Blood transfusion

Jehovah's Witnesses will not accept blood transfusion in any form. They will show many references from the Bible that the blood contains a man's soul. The soul is responsible for one's behaviour. Therefore giving blood from one person to another is taken to be transforming a person into another personality.

Where a Jehovah's Witness has to have a blood transfusion in a life-threatening situation, he will have a considerable guilt feeling. A GP should consider counselling in such a situation.

Plasma substitutes should be used wherever possible. Where a blood transfusion has to be given, a Jehovah's Witness priest should be consulted as, with other religions, the sanctity of life doctrine is practised by Jehovah's Witnesses. This doctrine states that killing is always wrong, no matter what the circumstances are. On this basis, a compromise can be reached.

Alcohol

In large amounts, alcohol affects a person's judgment. Therefore, Islam has emphatically prohibited its use. A Muslim patient should not be prescribed medicines containing alcohol, such as tonics and local antiseptics such as surgical spirit.

A patient may be too polite to point this out to the doctor, but not only will he not use the prescribed medication, but also he will tell other Muslim patients not to consult that particular doctor.

Some vegetarians, and especially vegans, will not accept eggs. Certain measles, influenza and yellow fever vaccines are prepared in egg medium. The patient is asked before their administration whether they are allergic to eggs. A vegetarian is usually a Hindu Gujarati Indian patient, and these are very polite people.

First published in *Pulse Reference Series*, **43**, Nov. 12, 1983 (Morgan Grampian Professional Press Ltd.)

They will leave your clinic or surgery, never to return, if offered such vaccines with such a query. Their children and elderly patients could be at risk from these illnesses, and should be under surveillance.

Pork

Religions always take something as a symbol. Islamic and Jewish religions have taken pork as a symbol of uncleanliness and insulins derived from pork are not acceptable to these patients. If a Muslim patient is allergic to beef and not allowed pork, he may be prescribed Humulin or Human insulin.

There is a problem here. The name 'Humulin' implies that it is derived from human flesh. A doctor should not take it for granted that patients are aware that these new insulins are synthetic and not derived from some animal source. He should, in fact, explain this to the patient before prescribing it. Pork insulin is allowed to Jews, but pork by mouth remains a strong taboo.

Beef

The cow is sacred to Hindus, who come mainly from India. The map of old India resembles the shape of the cow. They do not even like the cow to be called an animal because in their eyes an animal is lower in status than the cow.

For centuries, the cow, a family pet, was the source of milk for adults as well as children. Therefore beef insulin will not be accepted by Hindus. If they are allergic to pork insulin and have to have Humulin or Human insulin, they should be told that it is synthetic in origin, if it is so. Some Human insulins are derived from pork.

Uncircumcised males

Phimosis and paraphimosis used to be common illnesses in ancient times. Those were the days long before antiseptics were invented, let alone antibiotics.

Religion is responsible for the wellbeing of its followers and that includes their physical, psychological, social and financial wellbeing.

Female circumcision is not a religious custom.

Because male circumcision is not carried out under the National Health Service, this compulsory ritual has to be performed by private practitioners in this country and non-medical practitioners in the Asian subcontinent.

There was a time when abortion was performed by private practitioners and we called it 'back-street abortion'. To stop that illegal practice, abortion was legalised under the Abortion Act 1967. Perhaps the time has come to stop back-street circumcision and allow this operation to be performed under the NHS for Muslims and Jews.

Moral issues

Adherents of Judaism, Christianity, Islam, Hinduism and Buddhism will have strong and divergent views on abortion, contraception, infanticide, artificial insemination, test tube babies, suicide, euthanasia, burial and cremation.

All these should be considered when making a decision. For instance a Hindu British soldier who died in the Falklands was buried with other English soldiers. His family was greatly distressed because burial is not allowed in the Hindu religion. Hindus always cremate their dead.

Muslims, however, always bury their dead, and do not allow cremation. If the religious views of a patient are ignored, it can cause great anguish, which may not be revealed to the doctor.

COMMUNITY CONSIDERATIONS AND CONSULTATION

Social class/caste system

The caste system has existed in India since ancient times. Since 1921, the Registrar General of England has adopted the social class system. The caste system only applies to Hindus and is only adhered to in India. There are four castes:
–   Brahmins (high priests and the highest caste people)
–   Kshtriya (armed forces and civil servants)
–   Vaishya (business people)
–   Kshudra (untouchables – cleaners)
    This broadly corresponds to the social class system:
–   Professional
–   Intermediate
–   Skilled
–   Semi-skilled
–   Unskilled
    Both systems are based on one's occupation. One's social class can be altered but one's caste is permanent.

Panchayat (five wise men) system

This is practised among Asians. In the event of a dispute, civil or criminal, an out-of-Court discussion and settlement is reached in a meeting held by relatives and friends of both parties under the co-chairmanship of five persons that they all agree to trust. This ancient custom has been adopted by English courts in the form of the jury system. The medical profession has modified this to the 'three wise men' system.

A GP may find his ethnic minority patients turning to their own community for settlement of disputes where medico-legal reports are not necessary. This system can be used to decide non-accidental injury cases in high schools where the parties accept the headmaster, school medical officer, social worker and both parents as a 'panchayat'. Serious cases, of course, would have to be referred to the Law.

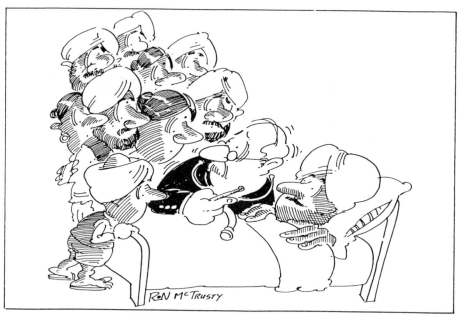

Don't be surprised by relatives and friends in the Asian 'open house' – they may want to monitor the GP's visit

Open house

In Eastern cultures, unexpected guests normally turn up without any warning and therefore families always cook large amounts of food to cope with such common occurences.

When a GP is visiting a house, he should not be surprised to see many relatives and friends by the bedside of the sick person. They may not, in fact, be overcrowding the accommodation and may only be visiting to monitor the GP's visit.

They might even ask the GP the nature and progress of the illness and its management because they believe in 'shared privacy'. An English GP needs to reconcile his own belief in confidentiality with this community approach.

DOES YOUR PATIENT SMOKE?

Chapter 7 mentioned the use of hooka pipes, but there are other sources of tobacco. If a GP asks some first generation Asians if they smoke they may well answer 'No' assuming that he is referring only to cigarettes. But they may smoke 'beedees' (Birix). These consist of tobacco rolled in a beedee leaf, and will be supplied by friends and relatives who visit Asia.

With the Sikh religion smoking is taboo and a Sikh patient will be offended if he is asked point blank whether he smokes. Perhaps this question should be posed indirectly, such as 'You are a Sikh. You don't smoke, do you?'

CULTURAL TABOOS

Health visitors and social workers

In an extended family, it is the responsibility of the grandparents to act as health visitors and social workers in the family, advising on infant feeding, shopping, marital problems, family frictions, schooling and cultural heritage.

If a health visitor or a social worker visits, for example, an Asian family, the neighbours come to ask the parents what the matter is. They have to explain to the neighbours because of shared responsibility, and it can cause embarrassment.

A health visitor, social worker, district nurse or a home help who telephones the family first and makes an appointment to visit them if necessary will establish a closer rapport with Eastern families. However, these families will be perfectly happy to attend the health centre for such consultations. A flexible attitude is desirable.

Sex education

In Eastern cultures and some religions, sex education in schools is strictly forbidden. The knowledge of the facts of life is passed on by a male family member to males, and by female family members to females, usually uncles or aunts.

Therefore, GPs and other members of the primary care team should be very cautious when handling this issue. Teenagers from ethnic minority groups already face the 'two-culture conflict'. Mishandling of this issue can have disastrous results, both for the teenager and the whole family.

PHYSICAL DIFFERENCES

Vision

Recent studies have suggested that early deterioration of visual acuity, especially for reading, is more common among ethnic Asians than other ethnic groups. It is said that those affected will need spectacles before the age of 40. However, this frequently occurs at a much earlier age, and particularly in childhood.

Most Asian parents blame this visual deterioration on watching television. Not only should they be counselled on this, but ethnic Asian school children should have more frequent vision tests by school nurses.

In such a child, apparent lack of progress at school may result, and their vision should be tested before they are referred to an educational psychologist.

Red cell sodium/potassium pump

In hypertensives, red cell sodium/potassium pump activity is increased. It has been noted that this only occurs in Europeans and no such difference was noted in Asian or Afro-Caribbean patients suffering from hypertension.

Haemolysis

Phenazone (antipyrine) is reported to cause haemolysis in glucose-6-PD-deficient Europeans, but not in glucose-6-PD-deficient Afro-Caribbeans.

There seems to be a scientific basis for carrying out more research in these areas because all patients from all ethnic groups cannot always have the same treatment.

DIET/DRUG INTERACTION

Drug activity

We are aware that normal drug activity differs, not only genetically, but also according to which ethnic group a patient belongs to. This can be measured by testing the 'acetylator status' – this is the rate at which a patient inactivates a drug by the acetylation process.

Phenelzine, sulphonamides and isoniazid are examples of drugs whose metabolism is found to differ in different races.

The clinical response to drugs, including adverse side-effects, will vary. Half the population of the UK and US are found to be slow metabolisers compared with 1% of Canadian Eskimos and 82% of Egyptians.

A patient with depression will improve more with phenelzine (MAOI) if he is a slow metaboliser but will have more side-effects such as postural hypotension. We are aware of numerous drug interactions, including MAOIs and some foods.

The MAOIs may cause a dangerous rise in blood pressure when interacting with tyramine-containing foods such as cheese, pickled herrings, broad bean pods, Bovril, Oxo, Marmite, yeast and Chianti wine. All these foods may be eaten by health food lovers.

Tandoori nan (an Indian food), which contains large amounts of yeast, is becoming popular in the UK.

Cough mixtures and decongestant nasal drops may contain sympatho-mimetic drugs. These may be bought over the counter. Their pressor action may be potentiated by MAOI compounds, resulting in a rise in blood pressure.

This may lead to a throbbing headache which is an early warning symptom. Further complications may follow. This example highlights drug – food interaction and is the tip of an iceberg.

Cabbage

This is said to contain an antithyroid agent. A patient with thyroid disorders should be asked about the amount of cabbage he is eating so that his therapy can be adjusted accordingly.

Rose hips

These are used in betel chewing. They contain 60 times more vitamin C than lemons. High doses of vitamin C can give a false negative result on Clinistix urine-testing, thereby masking a profound glycosuria. This is because the enzyme in Clinistix is inhibited by ascorbic acid. As a result, a diabetes mellitus may remain uncontrolled.

Milk

This is said to considerably reduce the therapeutic effectiveness of tetracyclines. A patient should be advised not to take this medication with milk, but to swallow the tablets with water.

These are just three of the numerous examples of diet – drug interactions.

COUNSELLING AND MANAGEMENT

Ethnic majority groups may be considered on the basis of an age and sex register, but for ethnic minority groups, in addition to this, we need to have a three-generation concept:
-   The first generation – retired people
-   Second generation – workers
-   Third generation – children and adolescents

A *patient from the first generation* when facing an English GP may experience colour shock. He may look away when he is talking to the GP as it is his cultural attitude. He may keep on nodding his head out of politeness, even if he does not understand what is being said. He may ask what food to avoid and put on a silent smile.

A British GP dealing with a first generation patient may find his name difficult to understand.

He may look right into the patient's eyes and explain the prescription as well as emphasising the compliance needed. He may use sign language. Unless patience, understanding and positive effort are exercised, the GP consultation may end up as a disaster. The GP may be amused or irritated, but such an ethnic minority patient goes home confused and bewildered.

A *second generation patient*, who is a worker, possibly in a factory or in a business, may visit the British GP with a two-culture conflict. He may be very angry if patronised by the GP. He will be very sensitive of any denigration, even if inadvertently expressed. Sometimes he may over-imitate and become more English than the English, or exercise his parents' culture more rigidly.

A GP dealing with such a patient should be very tactful, avoid denigration or patronisation, and with patience a good rapport can be established.

A *third generation ethnic minority group patient*, a school child or an adolescent, behaves more like his English counterpart. Although he will be less clear of his personal identity, he will use an English accent, will feel very British and present with English diseases.

In conclusion: recent research has shown that ethnic factors have a direct influence on health, disease and a doctor's management. A greater understanding and an effort to improve the situation will promote health and a GP is in a privileged position to take the initiative.

CHAPTER 10

ALTERNATIVE THERAPIES AND ETHNIC GROUPS

Different ethnic groups will have had varying degrees of exposure to and use of alternative therapies which are specific to their cultures, for example:

Ethnic Asians
  Hikmat
  Homoeopathy
  Ayurvedic
  Massage therapy
  Faith healing
  Religious therapy
  Folklore medicine
  Urinotherapy (Murarji Desai, former Prime Minister of India, used this therapy)
  Magic

Ethnic Chinese
  Acupuncture
  Zen (meditation with eyes open, popular among Buddhists)
  Faith healing (Buddhist)
  Folklore medicine (Chinese)

Ethnic Afro-Caribbeans
  Faith healing
  Religious therapy (Christian)
  Folklore medicine (tribal)

Continuing to use some of these therapies in parallel with GP dispensed services may result in some patients receiving 'multi-therapy' with potential hazard to the consumer.

Patients may receive 'alternative treatments' for anxiety states, tension, chronic pain, allergies, psychosomatic disorders, chronic diseases and terminal illnesses.

Europeans may be fond of health foods, herbal medicine and homoeopathic remedies, whereas non-Europeans may visit a 'Hakim' (a herbalist and dietician), an 'Ayurvedic practitioner' (elemental therapist), a faith healer, or may

First published in *Pulse Reference Series*, **43**, Nov. 12, 1983 (Morgan Grampian Professional Press Ltd.)

even be undergoing acupuncture or urinotherapy. Moreover, Yoga and Transcendental Meditation may be practised daily.

Some dangerous drugs may be bought over the counter on holidays abroad. Patients may not necessarily tell their GP about this – they only tell their doctors what they think he wants to hear.

Some patients, however, have communication difficulties with their doctors on account of a 'social class barrier'. They may conceal such facts in order to avoid annoying him.

Specifics

There may be specific problems with specific remedies.

Homoeopathic remedies

A patient with hay fever may use 'combination I' tablets (homoeopathic remedy). He may then come with ocular and nasal symptoms to his GP, who prescribes eyedrops and a nasal spray. He will refuse to take antihistamine tablets as he is already taking 'combination I' tablets. The result will be partial compliance. One would never know which therapy is the successful one.

Hakim's medicine

A Hakim may prescribe a 'mercury kusta' (an aphrodisiac) to a patient over a long period. He may develop mercury psychosis (mad as a hatter) and may thus consult the GP, who could remain unaware of the reason for his behaviour.

Specific foods

Drugs can also interact with specific foods used by different cultures. For example, an Indian vegetable 'karela' (*Mormordica charantia*) potentiates chlorpropamide; this can induce a prolonged state of hypoglycaemia. It is of interest that Hakims use karela powder in order to treat diabetes mellitus. Moreover, karela curry is becoming an increasingly popular dish in the UK.

In addition, some foods may cause allergy. Practitioners of alternative medicine generally advise some form of dietary restriction.

Drugs bought abroad

When on holiday abroad, a patient may buy 'Cibalgin' for relief of pain, and suffer dental damage as a consequence. The use of Enterovioform for travellers' diarrhoea may lead to paralysis of the legs or optic atrophy. An infant may be given 'Lactogen' (baby milk) and may develop 'bottle baby disease'.

Such drugs are banned in the UK but sold over the counter in Third World countries. On return to this country, the patient may seek the advice of his GP regarding side-effects although he may conceal the name of the actual drug in order to avoid embarrassment. Remedies or other therapies may be purchased in the same way, which may cause adverse side-effects.

The result as far as the GP is concerned is that his patient would present problems of non-compliance or partial compliance. A drug given to a patient receiving multiple therapies could be potentiated or may interact or counteract with another remedy prescribed.

Illegal drugs

In medicine 'one can never say never and never say always because there is always an exception to the rule'. Similarly a patient may be using an illegal drug and deny the fact point-blank. A GP may find it more helpful to look for signs rather than symptoms of a suspected case.

An illegal drug may be opium, LSD, cannabis, heroin or cocaine. One should bear in mind the following possibilities:

–   An interaction between a GP-prescribed medicine and hard drugs. For example, opium or morphine may interact with MAOIs.
–   The objective evidence of withdrawal symptoms or signs of toxicity of the drugs of addiction.
–   Nutritional deficiencies which may result.
–   The anxiety of the patient with regard to a doctor's confidentiality. He watches TV where he sees so much debate on computerised personal data and the risk to an individual's confidentiality.

Health foods and medicine

A diabetic patient may be taking health food (medicine) with a high vitamin C content (500 mg daily, or more). He may have a false negative result on a urine test for glucose with Clinistix, while he may in fact have profound glycosuria. This is because the enzyme in the Clinistix is inhibited by the ascorbic acid. As a result the diabetes mellitus may remain uncontrolled.

Part II
SPECIAL
CONSIDERATIONS

Note: Each chapter in this section was originally written for a different audience, as commissioned by the editors of the various journals, therefore, in order to keep each chapter complete in itself, some repetition is inevitable.

CHAPTER 11

CULTURAL CONFLICTS IN A MIXED MARRIAGE

Mixed marriages are becoming increasingly common in the UK and present their own special problems and opportunities for misunderstanding. Although no GP wants to spend too much time acting as a marriage counsellor, it is to him or her that these difficulties may first become apparent disguised as a medical problem.

This chapter outlines some of the cultural conflicts whithin mixed marriages of which the GP should be aware.

This chapter is intended to help GPs play a positive role in helping mixed marriage families, with physical, psychological, social, sexual and cultural difficulties that can arise.

In the UK there are three models: 'marriage between equals', 'father and mother roles' and 'mother and father roles'.

– 'Marriage between equals' is more popular among the British. Both partners share wage earnings and domestic tasks. The economic necessities of modern life have made them adopt this style or marriage. Women's Liberation is the cause as well as the effect.

– 'Father and mother roles' are adhered to by ethnic Asians. The father is the wage earner and the mother plans how to spend the money. This is due to the influence of religions.

– 'Mother and father roles' are common in ethnic Afro-Caribbeans. The mother leads the family.

There are, of course, many exceptions to these broadly-based categories, depending on many variables.

TWO-CULTURE MARRIAGE

This seems to be a more appropriate description of the so-called 'mixed marriage'. Broadly speaking, there are two cultures in the world, Eastern and Western. However, there can be many subcultures.

Eastern behaviour is consistent with religious thinking, which is theoretical, empirical, moral and emotional.

Western behaviour is based on the scientific approach, which is practical, analytical, rational and unemotional.

First published in *Pulse Reference Series*, **45**, Jan. 26, 1985 (Morgan Grampian Professional Press Ltd.)

This difference of wavelength may lead to marital pathology. However, conflict can be avoided by making a positive effort to understand each other.

Physical differences

Let us assume that by a 'mixed marriage' we mean that one partner is ethnic English and the other is of non-English origin, and consider some examples.
- *Different eye colour.* A girl aged seven who had an Italian brown-eyed father and an English blue-eyed mother was brought to the GP because she had one brown eye and the other blue. The parents were worried in case she had some eye disease. Although the GP reassured them, when the child grows up she is more likely to develop 'heat cataract' in the blue eye than the brown.
- *Freckle clusters.* An infant who had an Iranian father and a red-headed Irish mother and was brought to the GP because he was born with large clusters of freckles all over his body, which they feared were some sinister disease. After consultation with a dermatologist, this was found to be physiological.
- *Cross-traits.* Disseminated sclerosis is more common among Europeans, thalassaemia is more predominant in Mediterraneans, and Afro-Caribbeans have a genetic predisposition to hypertension. Such hereditary disorders could be handed down to the child of mixed parentage. Perhaps a GP should tactfully ask the ethnic origin of the other partner.

Psychological problems

Marital stress is a common entity even in one-culture marriages but in mixed marriages some additional factors can lead to a breakdown unless recognised and dealt with sympathetically.

Fear of the unknown. Although most people marry the partner of their choice, when marrying into another culture or ethnic group it is natural to have some misgivings such as mistrust and misunderstanding, even if one does not admit it openly, which can lead to mishandling of certain situations. Where a communication barrier exists, a GP can help both partners to have a frank dialogue, leading to mutual understanding.

Stress from in-laws. Prejudices are part of human nature and race, culture and religion are no exceptions. If an English girl wants to marry a West Indian man, for instance, her family may do everything in their power to dissuade her.

In fact this pressure may make her over-react and force her into the marriage, and to make matters worse the family may disown the girl.

On the other hand, a West Indian migrant, who already has enough of his own problems, could be frightened off by the whole situation! If such a couple still gets married, the emotional tug-of-war may continue even after children are born, leading to severe psychological stress. Such a family may be frequent attenders at a surgery for many minor complaints which are really a 'cry for help'.

Social stigma. As with an unmarried mother, a mixed marriage is often regarded as a disgrace in some closed communities such as English villages. If a mixed-marriage couple move from a big city to the countryside, they and their children may face open hostility and their children may be victimised in schools. A country GP should be aware of this possibility.

Emotional frustration. An English partner may feel superior, an Asian man may try to dominate, an Afro-Caribbean woman will expect to be the decision-maker in her family, and a Vietnamese man may develop an inferiority complex if his English wife behaves in a superior manner.

Some people may have a higher expectation of a mixed marriage than a one-culture marriage, but when faced with the same financial and environmental obstacles, their disappointment will be greater under these circumstances. One or both partners may feel utterly frustrated and blame the mixed marriage for all their problems.

However, some couples may accept this challenge and strengthen their marriage.

Social issues

In most English marriages both partners go out to work, at least until children are born, in an attempt to meet the rising cost of living. However, in a mixed marriage a husband from an Eastern culture, especially a Muslim, expects his wife to stay at home – although few English women would be prepared to observe purdah!

Economic hardship. In Eastern cultures, based on the extended family system, the man has to support his dependent relatives in their country of origin for life. His English wife, having to stay at home, may choose to have more children for company. The husband's salary may not be sufficient to pay all the bills and expenses. This situation may result in frequent visits to the surgery with psychosomatic illnesses.

Marriages of convenience. Some partners marry for migration and nationality purposes, and having achieved this, they may find they have nothing in common with their spouses, and the marriage will fail.

Regular family visits. An Eastern man may visit his relatives living in the UK regularly, without his wife. Similarly, the English wife may visit her parents alone, if they disapprove of her marriage into another culture. This pattern could result in considerable marital disharmony.

Sexual difficulties

Sexual counsellors are well aware of difficulties in any marriage. However, in a mixed marriage some additional factors can be encountered which the partners, possibly due to cultural shyness, are unable to discuss between themselves, but would confide in a sympathetic GP.

Pubic hair. Shaving of the pubic hair by both men and women is an Eastern custom. Depilatory creams and soaps are widely available in Eastern countries. An English partner may be put off by this custom and similarly, an Eastern partner will be turned off by the presence of pubic hair. A simple explanation is all that is necessary.

Elixir of life. Hindu men, especially athletes, grow up with the belief that semen is the elixir of life and therefore may avoid intercourse, and this can be regarded as an insult by an English wife.

Headache. A Western wife may frequently complain of headaches when she does not feel like having sex. An Asian husband will be totally unaware of this excuse and may call the doctor.

Lovemaking. An Eastern man prefers to lie on top of his wife, placing a towel underneath her, switching the light off, and will not expect her to participate actively. However, a Western wife will not like to be a passive partner, may prefer the light to be on with soft music in the background, may not bother with a towel, and at times would like a change in position.

An English partner believes in foreplay and spends some time in 'after-play', and tries to ensure orgasm for both him and his wife. In keeping with the Eastern 'sex is taboo' attitude, an Eastern couple may consider love-making for procreation only and the importance of sexual pleasure may be underplayed. An Eastern woman may be happy to play a passive role and please her husband, and is not bothered about achieving an orgasm. This lack of active participation may lead to failure of erection, a common complaint in Eastern men.

The irony of this is that the *Kama Sutra* was the first book on sexology in the world, written by a Hindu, but the author was never popular in his life-time!

Kissing. Passionate kissing in Western cultures means kissing lip-to-lip, but in the East this is never done. Couples kiss each other lip-to-cheek and it is not uncommon to see a love-bite on the cheek of a European wife or an Eastern husband. Such a wife may consult her GP, thinking she has halitosis, because she is too shy to ask her husband frankly why he does not kiss her on the lips.

Incidentally, the GP may notice teeth-marks on her cheek, especially the left cheek, and may suspect wife-beating. In fact, it is a cross-cultural love bite.

Communication barriers

Small talk. British couples chat over the day's events and domestic matters, especially about their pets and children. This small talk is not appreciated by an Eastern husband or wife because they are used to speaking about important points only and adhere rigidly to the dictum 'think before you speak'.

An English doctor sometimes likes to chat to his patients before the actual consultation. An English wife will appreciate this, but her Eastern husband may be annoyed at what he thinks is a waste of time.

Difference of opinion. An English husband expects an Asian wife to have her own opinion and not necessarily to agree with him all the time, but she, being brought up in a culture where a difference of opinion is not allowed, may tend to agree with him all the time because to her a difference of opinion invites some form of punishment.

Language traps. In some Eastern languages there are no such words as 'please' or 'the', and politeness is expressed by gesture and the tone of the voice. A Western wife will be offended when a Sikh husband appears to give orders to her, which are, in fact, intended as polite requests.

Time to speak. In Eastern cultures the elderly have the right to speak before others and they believe that age brings wisdom and that they are always right. In an extended family, the mother or father-in-law dominates the whole family.

At a dining table, even with invited guests, an Asian host may unwittingly behave like a chairman and determine who should speak first and what topics should be discussed. A Christmas party in such a family can be a traumatic experience.

Different meanings. Some everyday gestures have very different meanings in different cultures. For example the 'thumbs up' sign used by the British to indicate success is, in fact, a rude gesture to a Belgian, Greek or Cypriot. Hence when an English husband and Greek wife visited a Scottish GP to consult about their son, and he reassured them about their child's health by raising his thumb, the wife was very upset.

Obviously, there are many such examples in verbal and non-verbal communication where problems arise between two cultures.

Uneasy silence. An Eastern person likes constant conversation and does not appreciate periods of silence which are culturally part of the English way of relaxation and this can also cause problems in a multi-cultural social gathering. The English wife may be quietly and happily observing her surroundings and the people around her, but her Asian husband may feel embarrassed at this and may tell her to speak. This may be a useful point to bear in mind in marital counselling.

Uneasy truce. Due to language barriers, a mixed marriage couple may not be open with each other because some important and intimate matters may be too complicated for translation, and may resort to trivia to hide any embarrassment. This can cause severe communication breakdown.

Religious matters

Jews. It has been said that as many as 33 per cent of the Jews in this country marry outside their faith, and this is frowned upon by orthodox Jews and can cause severe conflicts within a family. This, of course, can also apply to devout Muslims, Hindus, Sikhs, Catholics and Buddhists.

Catholics. Contraception, pre-marital sex and abortion are strongly condemned among Catholics. This may cause considerable stress in a marriage between a Catholic and, for example, a Hindu.

The Catholic Church only allows a mixed marriage on condition that the children are brought up in the Catholic faith.

For example, a Catholic girl married a Muslim and had a son and daughter. The husband planned a holiday in the south of France after selling the house in England with a view to buying another one. He disappeared without notice with the children and was later found to have returned to Pakistan, leaving his Catholic wife behind. To a Muslim, it causes great distress to see his daughter being brought up as a non-Muslim and not wearing purdah. However, he would be more tolerant where his son is concerned.

If these religious convictions are discussed before the mixed marriage takes place, such heartbreak can be avoided.

A GP should realise that it is not just a matter of a father running away with the children, it is the result of a clash between two strong religious doctrines.

Muslims. A devout Muslim is expected to have a shower after sex and will expect his wife to do the same, especially early in the morning before the time of morning prayer. In overcrowded accommodation this can cause embarrassment, the wife may make excuses not to make love and the husband may consult his doctor about her alleged frigidity.

Circumcision is a religious custom for Muslims and Jews and such wives may have reservations about marrying an uncircumcised man. Nevertheless, an Eastern woman, because of cultural shyness, may never look at her husband's genitalia!

Taboos. Alcohol is forbidden to Muslims and smoking is taboo to Sikhs. An English wife may drink or smoke in secret, and when caught, her husband may accuse her of being an alcoholic and suspect other vices, and may seek the help of his doctor.

Cultural conflicts

Hygiene. The English often use a handbasin filled with water for washing their faces and other parts of the body, enjoy a good long soak in a hot bath, and use toilet paper after defaecation. On the other hand, Asian and Chinese wash their faces under running water, enjoy a shower, disliking the idea of sitting in used water, and always wash after defaecation, whether they use paper or not.

In the UK, where toilet facilities do not include water for washing, and an Eastern-type water container is not available, an Asian will use any suitable container for water, even an empty milk bottle! Not only will the milkman be short of empty bottles as a result, but the English wife and children will wonder what on earth their father wants with an empty milk bottle in the lavatory!

An Asian husband may consider his wife unhygienic and similarly an English wife may blame him, and this matter can eventually reach the GP.

Family outings. An English husband will often try to avoid crowds, find a secluded spot on the beach, or drive to a quiet part of the countryside, whereas his Eastern wife may prefer to take the children shopping or to a crowded funfair. Unless there is a compromise, such a family could end up spending their leisure hours separately.

Pocket money. An English mother may allow her children to spend their pocket money as they wish, whereas her Asian husband expects them to save their money because he is concerned with their future interests rather than their wishes.

Toys or food. An Asian mother buys extra food for her children rather than toys. Some such children may not even have seen building bricks or Ladybird books and may fail the developmental examination at the GP surgery. An English father, on the other hand, buys toys for his children and even plays with them himself!

Punishment. The English have a personality profile – vision, hearing and touch. But the Continentals and non-Europeans have the personality profile – touch, hearing and vision.

It is not uncommon for an Asian or West Indian husband to hit his wife or children and within their culture this is acceptable. Many English health visitors and school-teachers will be up in arms when they find a schoolchild with a bruise during physical education classes and will call a case conference. This distresses the whole family.

If the GP has a quiet word with the husband or father and explains that this is unacceptable in this country, he will co-operate.

Remarriage. Divorce is frowned upon in all religions and many cultures. For Catholics it is taboo and considered a stigma by Asians. An Asian man will be very reluctant to marry a divorcee, and if he does marry her, will hide this fact from his relatives and friends.

Christians and Muslims believe in remarriage but Hindus have many reservations about it.

Household pets. The English like a cat or a dog in the house, whereas Asians will not allow this because they are brought up to believe that dogs, particularly, are dirty and untouchable. They would prefer to have a cow or a goat as a pet, although this would be rather difficult in a city!

Birthdays and death days. Birthdays are celebrated in the West, but not in the East, where only prophets' and saints' birthdays are celebrated. Even now, in some parts of India births are not registered.

Therefore a great problem arises when a GP receptionist asks for an Asian patient's date of birth when that patient may not even know his own age. If he marries a European, his wife may suspect him of concealing his real age, because age is so important in the west.

Forty-day rule. In Asian cultures, when a child is born the mother is not allowed to set foot outside her house for 40 days, not even to see the GP. Similarly, a widow is not allowed to go out, even to visit the doctor, for 40 days after the death of her husband. They are looked after by the relatives in the extended family system.

This means that the GP may be asked to make housecalls if such a woman needs help. This may be considered unnecessary by the English relatives or doctors. A sympathetic understanding is essential.

Rebound marriages. If a mixed marriage fails, the partners may blame each other's culture and vow never to marry outside their own culture again, and may develop a pathological hatred of the former partner's culture. Such past experiences could be one of the reasons for racial prejudice.

Virginity. An Eastern man expects his wife to be a virgin and may feel very guilty if he marries a European following pre-marital sex. This guilt feeling may lead him to consult.

Correct terminology

'Half-caste' is a term which should never be used, especially in front of the children of mixed marriages. It is the most insulting name they could be called – even worse than 'bastard'. This term originated because there was an absolute taboo on cross-cultural marriages and it was used as a form of abuse.

Nowadays, with the increase in understanding and financial interdependence between cultures, people do not fear intermarrying. The children of such a marriage can be referred to as children of mixed parentage and this can be further qualified by mentioning the ethnic origin of each parent, e.g. if a father is English and a mother Chinese, the child will be Anglo-Chinese.

However, there is one exception and that is Anglo-Indian. This term has been commonly used for Christian Indians and does not signify that one parent was English and the other Indian. In fact, there were very few mixed marriages in this subculture. Where one parent is English and the other Indian, the accepted term is 'Eurasian'.

Similarly, Asians, especially Sri Lankans, hate to be called 'black', and dislike the term 'coloured'. However, they are quite happy with 'dark-skinned' or 'brown', or even 'tropical colour'.

Of course, Europeans are happy to be called 'white' and Afro-Caribbeans believe that 'black is beautiful'. Nevertheless, Chinese do not like to be called 'yellow' and prefer 'light-skinned'.

CHAPTER 12

DISEASE PATTERNS IN VARIOUS ETHNIC GROUPS IN THE UNITED KINGDOM

If someone copies from one author it is labelled as plagiarism but if someone copies from more than one author it is called research. This chapter is a 1994 update of the research evidence available on medical problems encountered in various ethnic groups in the UK. For the sake of brevity, only those diseases are mentioned here which may be of practical value to a practising doctor and the account is kept short enough to be informative as well as entertaining. However, a list of references is provided for those who wish to pursue topics in greater depth.

In the practice of medicine, it is useful to learn about the natural history of a disease and to construct a profile of a typical patient. However, a profile should not be mistaken for stereotyping which is a negative concept. When a doctor diagnoses a squint or epilepsy he or she wants to help the patient and it should not be interpreted as stigmatisation. Although any disease can occur in almost every ethnic group, there are certain diseases which are more predominant in a particular ethnic population. Consequently, it is prudent to be aware of the disease patterns of various groups and this awareness can be of clinical value for an accurate diagnosis and also for planning services to meet appropriate health needs of all ethnic groups.

ETHNIC EUROPEANS

Denis Burkitt coined the term 'Western diseases' after a life of research and listed the diseases which are more common among Europeans when compared with Asians and Africans. Western diseases fall into four categories[1]:
A. Cardiovascular diseases such as coronary heart disease, hypertension, cerebrovascular disease, peripheral vascular disease, and varicose veins.
B. Gastrointestinal diseases such as appendicitis, constipation, diverticular disease, haemorrhoids, colonic cancer and polyps, hiatus hernia, coeliac disease, and Crohn's disease.
C. Metabolic disorders such as diabetes (mature onset), obesity, hyper-uricaemia, and gout.
D. Miscellaneous diseases such as pernicious anaemia, multiple sclerosis, thyrotoxicosis, dental caries, gall stones, renal stones, and, of course, chronic bronchitis – the English disease.

Social drinking and going to the pub are ingrained in the fabric of the Western culture but alcoholism is another matter. "Alcohol . . . provokes the desire but takes away the performance" (Macbeth). Alcoholism is the fifth most common cause of death in the UK. It can lead to malnutritional anaemias, social deterioration, loss of job, marital breakdown, and makes a person prone to accidents. It is an occupational hazard of pub landlords.

English studies identify that the Irish drink most and the Irish authors go to town in writing that the English drink the most. The French tease the Scots for drunkenness and vice versa. Nevertheless, whisky drinking is more common in Ireland, Scotland and England. The French drink more wine than spirits. Alcoholism also affects religious ceremonies, e.g. in Sligo, Ireland, on Christmas Eve, midnight mass in churches is held at 10.00 pm for obvious reasons.

A non-European doctor, particularly someone from a culture where alcohol is forbidden, should show respect to a European patient's social drinking and also remain sympathetic in the management of alcoholism.

Ethnic English, Scottish, and Welsh – In addition to Western diseases, recent evidence suggests that some conditions are more common in these ethnic majority groups (see Table 1).

Table 1. Diseases: Ethnic connection

Ethnic group	Disease
English	Cystic fibrosis, pernicious anaemia
Irish	Lung cancer, tuberculosis
Jewish	Tay – Sachs disease, Niemann – Pick disease
Italians	Congenital hip dislocation
Asians	Lactose intolerance, rickets, tuberculosis
Afro-Caribbeans	Catarrhal child syndrome, hernias (e.g. umbilical)

Pernicious anaemia is the most common cause of Vitamin B_{12} deficiency in UK whites and it is rare in Africans and Asians[2]. Cystic fibrosis, phenylketonuria, homocystinuria and spinal muscular atrophy (Werding Hoffman disease) are more common in whites than non-whites in the UK and these are autosomal recessive conditions[3].

Fuller and Toon[4] emphasise that multiple sclerosis, breast cancer, and inflammatory bowel disease are common among the British whites and rare in British Asians and British Africans/Caribbeans.

Rhesus incompatibility occurs when the infant is Rh-positive and the mother is Rh-negative. About 15% of caucasian women are Rh-negative whereas only 1% of black mothers are Rh-negative. This ethnic difference accounts for the greatly reduced incidence of rhesus incompatibility among the black population[5]. Other figures for Rh-negative women are 15% in Americans, 10% in Pakistanis and North Indians, 5% in South Indians, and only 1% in Chinese and South-East Asians. The proportion of Rh-negative people diminishes the nearer one gets to East and South-East Asia[6].

Any candidate taking the MRCGP or other professional examination must recite to the examiners three magic words – physical, psychological, and social (aspects of disease) – and remember that the most common causes of ill health and death in British whites are: coronary heart disease among middle-aged men[7]; breast cancer in women; cancer of other parts of the body in the elderly; accidents in school children; and congenital abnormalities in the newborn. Recently, the incidence of acquired immune deficiency has increased.

However, if the examiners are willing to listen or ask then the candidate should also mention the disease pattern in other ethnic groups and the findings, such as non-white children have grey reflex and not red reflex in the eyes.

Ethnic Irish – Irish people in Britain have a higher mortality rate than the English and Welsh from almost every cause of death except multiple sclerosis, diabetes mellitus, and carcinoma of the breast and uterus. They have, particularly, a higher mortality from tuberculosis and lung cancer (this is also prevalent in ethnic Scots). The prevalence of heavy smoking (20 or more cigarettes a day) is also higher among the Irish[8].

Ethnic French, Germans, Spanish, and Americans – Interestingly, the belief about the prevalence of a certain disease may be a central point in one nation's profile but it may be considered an exaggeration or non-disease by another nation. This contradiction of views affects both the patient and the doctor alike. Let us take four examples:

1. The English are brought up to take a keen interest in the regularity and consistency of their bowel movements. A preoccupation with bowel disorders lasts for life. An English person will see the doctor often with the complaint of constipation, and later laxative-induced looseness, and ask for oral medication[9].

2. The French, understandably, given their eating and drinking habits, view every ailment as a by-product of liver dysfunction. The cure for everything, therefore, is to drink more Badoit, Evian, and Perrier. If this fails, the entire system has to be purged by the French panacea – suppositories[10].

3. Virtually all Germans have health problems and if they don't there must be something wrong with them. They blame all ailments on disruption of the circulation such as cardiac insufficiency and low blood pressure. It is safer to steal a lioness' cub than to come between a German and his medication[11].

4. The Spanish are fascinated by their blood. Some Spaniards like visiting the doctor and others fear to do so. They often visit a pharmacist for pills and tonics[12].

A medical diagnosis can also be influenced by the cultural background of the doctor. For example, a patient with vague digestive troubles, where organic cause has been ruled out, can be diagnosed by: an American doctor as a food allergy; a British doctor as a virus infection; a French physician as a liver crisis; and by a German physician as a weak heart or low blood pressure[13].

ETHNIC ASIANS

A sensitive author feels obliged to respond positively to readers' feedback. The first edition of this book was reviewed by 22 medical journals in the UK. One objection across the board was the repetition of some facts throughout the text. Where possible, I have tried to redress the balance.

Asians make the second largest population in the world after Chinese and they are the largest ethnic minority group in the UK. The diseases which are common in this group include: rickets (pp. 181, 189); osteomalacia (pp. 94, 181); haemoglobinopathy D – Punjab disease (pp. 15, 59); iron deficiency anaemia (pp. 25, 181); oral cancer (pp. 65, 213); tuberculosis (pp. 35, 86, 207); malaria (pp. 86, 93); amoebic dysentery (pp. 35, 87); and typhoid (p. 35, 165).

Recent evidence[14] suggests two significant findings:

1. According to a Leicestershire study there appears to be more than an expected occurrence amongst Asians of cancers of the tongue, oral cavity, pharynx, oesophagus and of some other sites when compared with English patients. The excess of Asian cancer cases at particular sites found in the study was attributed to the Asian habit of betel chewing.

2. Tuberculosis was a killer disease in the UK and it was often referred to as the 'white man's plague'. Bunyan, in his writings, labelled it as 'Captain of the men of death'. In 1855, for example, 13% of deaths from all causes were attributed to tuberculosis but in the early 1990s the figure has fallen to 0.1%. However, immigrant groups are more prone to tuberculosis for a number of reasons. It is not surprising that respiratory tuberculosis is three times more common among the Irish and 30 times more common in ethnic Asians. Non-pulmonary tuberculosis is 80 times more common among those of Asian origin than the English population. Nevertheless, the situation is expected to improve with time if appropriate steps are taken.

ETHNIC JEWS

Tay – Sachs disease and Niemann – Pick disease are both common in infants of Jewish origin (p. 14). Tay – Sachs disease is 100 times more likely to occur in a Jewish couple than in a non-Jewish couple and 85% of babies born with this disease are Jewish because the carrier state for this condition in North and East European Jews is 1 in 25 whereas it is 1 in 250 among the white British population[4]. A doctor should contact the Tay – Sachs Society in London (Tel: 081-550-8989) for advice.

ETHNIC ARABS

Bilharziasis (schistosomiasis) is a condition in which a patient may pass blood in his or her urine without pain. Many Arabs visit their homeland on holiday and the Nile is heavily infected with *Schistosoma haematobium*. This condition is endemic in Egypt and also found in Iraq, Syria, Iran, Saudi Arabia, the Lebanon, the Yemen, the east coast of Africa, Israel, Turkey and Cyprus.

Another type of this disease occurs in China, Japan, Vietnam, the Phillipines, Laos and Thailand. An ethnic point to remember is that if a patient presents with painless haematuria, the most likely cause in an Englishman would be cancer of the bladder; in an ethnic Asian it may be tuberculosis of the kidney; and in an ethnic Arab it could be bilharziasis. An accurate diagnosis can save lives.

Carcinoma of the thyroid is said to be more common in some endemic areas of the world, especially Kuwait.

ETHNIC AFRICANS AND CARIBBEANS

The most significant medical conditions prevalent among this second largest ethnic minority group in Britain include sickle cell disease (pp. 15, 95), haemoglobinopathy C (pp. 15, 95), glucose-6-PD deficiency (pp. 15, 64), severe hypertension (pp. 12, 187), pill-induced hypertension (pp. 97, 115), hydroceles (pp. 15, 34), and hernias (pp. 34, 126).

As with ethnic Asians, ethnic Africans as well as Caribbean children normally have enlarged neck glands because their lymphoid tissue and skeletal tissue is more advanced at birth than ethnic Europeans. This ethnic gap is narrowed as the children grow older. Some European authors consider this lymphoid hyperplasia to be due to recurrent upper respiratory tract infection because catarrhal child syndrome is said to be more common in these children, perhaps due to the anatomical difference of the nasal sinuses.

After my talk to the GP trainees at the Whipps Cross Hospital (London) in 1992, two women GP trainees informed me that African and Caribbean children have grey reflex and not the red reflex which is present in European children's eyes. This is a point worth remembering in child surveillance clinics.

ETHNIC CYPRIOTS, GREEKS, AND TURKS

The commonest medical condition in these ethnic groups is beta-thalassaemia (pp. 14, 95), and iron therapy is contraindicated. The frequency of disease is 1 in 150 and of the carrier state is 1 in 6.

ETHNIC JAPANESE

Two common conditions are cancer of the stomach and a specific type of peptic ulcer (post-bulbar duodenal ulcer). Cancer of the stomach has been attributed to environmental factors such as the ingestion of raw fish, elements in water, and special methods of food preparation.

Post-bulbar duodenal ulcer – according to Western radiologists – is encountered in rice-eating populations such as the Japanese, Chinese, Bangladeshis, South Indians, and Sri Lankans. The husk of the rice becomes lodged in the posterior duodenal wall giving rise to this condition.

Such an ethnic minority patient who presents with simple indigestion over a period of time should be investigated with these possibilities in mind.

ETHNIC CHINESE

Their medical conditions include haemoglobinopathy E disease (pp. 15, 95). alpha-thalassaemia (pp. 15, 16), and the 'Chinese Restaurant Syndrome' (pp. 22, 68). In 1997 Hong Kong will be handed over to China and more Chinese are expected to arrive in Britain.

ETHNIC VIETNAMESE, MALAYS, INDONESIANS, THAIS AND FILIPINOS

In addition to alpha-thalassaemia, these ethnic groups from South-East Asia are likely to present with another form of bilharzia (*S. japanicum*). The bowel symptoms and barium enema appearances of *S. japanicum* infection may resemble those of amoebiasis or cancer of the colon.

CONCLUSION

An overview of multi-ethnic health issues has been briefly presented here, but there is more to it than meets the eye, and hopefully this chapter should whet the reader's appetite.

FURTHER READING

1. Burkitt, D. (1984). Dietary fibre – A way of preventing Western diseases. In: Pereira Gray, D.J. (ed.) *The Medical Annual*, Bristol: Wright, pp. 17–26
2. Jenkins, G.C. (1989). The blood. In: Swash, M. (ed.) *Hutchinson's Clinical Methods*, 19th edn., London: Bailliere Tindall, pp. 476–477
3. Blundy, S. (1985). Genetic disorders. In: Harvey, D. and Kovar, I. (eds) *Child Health*, Edinburgh: Churchill Livingstone, pp. 106–108
4. Fuller, J.H.S. and Toon, P.D. (1988). *Medical Practice in a Multicultural Society*. Oxford: Heinemann Professional, pp. 135–136 and 156–160
5. Jolly, H. and Levene, M. (1985). *Diseases of Children*, 5th edn., Oxford: Blackwell, pp. 111–115
6. Lewellyn-Jones, D. (1986). *Fundamentals of Obstetrics and Gynaecology, Vol. I. Obstetrics*, 4th edn., London: Faber and Faber, pp. 366–171
7. Editorial (1993). Health of the nation: calculating targets for coronary heart disease and stroke. *Br. J. Cardiol.*, **1(1)**, 11–12
8. Adelstein, A.M. and Marmot, M.G. (1989). The health of migrants in England and Wales: causes of death. In: Cruickshank, J. and Beevers, D.G. (eds.), *Ethnic Factors in Health and Disease*, London: Wright, pp. 43–47
9. Miall, A. (1993). *The Xenophobe's Guide to the English*, London: Ravette Books, pp. 45–46
10. Yapp, N. and Syrett, M. (1993). *The Xenophobe's Guide to the French*, London: Ravette Books, pp. 46–47
11. Zeidenitz, S. and Barkow, B. (1993). *The Xenophobe's Guide to the Germans*, London: Ravette Books, pp. 47–50
12. Lannay, D. (1993). *The Xenophobe's Guide to the Spanish*, London: Ravette Books, pp. 45–7
13. Payer, L. (1989). *Medicine and Culture*, London: Victor Gollancz, pp. 23–34
14. Donaldson, R.J. and Donaldson, L.J. (1993). *Essential Public Health Medicine*, Lancaster: Kluwer Academic Publishers, pp. 44–45 and 55–56

CHAPTER 13

HIDDEN CORNERS OF ETHNIC MEDICAL HISTORY

Transcultural medicine comprises encounters between a doctor of one ethnic group and his patient of another. The issues involved are medical (physical, psychological and social), religious, ethnic and cultural. There are hidden corners of ethnic medical history which have to be sought actively by the doctor if diagnostic traps are to be prevented. For example, a Welsh GP may move to England, believing that in this way he will improve 'sense' on both sides of the border. When treating a diabetic, he will determine the appropriate timing of his insulin or hypoglycaemic therapy, but, if he moves again to Scotland, he will have to change these timings because of the Scottish custom of 'high tea' instead of the English custom of 'dinner'.

In this short chapter I shall outline those specific hidden corners concerning ethnic groups which I have noted during my research in this area and medical observations over the last twenty years in London.

ETHNIC EUROPEANS

Hidden dangers of sliced bread plastic clips

The invention of plastic wrapping and plastic clips for packaged, sliced bread is the latest thing that has happened since the invention of sliced bread – another boon for the busy modern housewife! Unfortunately, when the sleepy housewife makes sandwiches early in the morning for her husband's lunch, it is possible for one such plastic clip to be accidentally included, and even eaten unnoticed by her husband at a hurried working lunch!

Recent correspondence in the *British Medical Journal* has reported some such cases where the clip has become embedded, gripping the bowel wall in between its 'jaws', and was becoming surrounded by an inflammatory mass. In addition to the risk of small bowel and oesophageal perforation, the symptoms of peptic ulcer may also be aggravated. The common symptoms could be stabbing epigastric pain at night, relieved by food. Some authorities have suggested that the white plastic clips could be replaced by larger, brightly-coloured or radio-opaque clips. However, this rarity should be borne in mind if the gastro-intestinal symptoms persist[1].

The material was first published in *J. Roy. Soc. Health*, **106**, No.5, Oct. 1986, pp.185 – 187 (Royal Society of Health)

Nicotine chewing gum

In smoking clinics, in addition to acupuncture, aversion therapy, group therapy and hypnosis, the use of nicotine chewing gum is being strongly advocated[2]. This gum is available in two strengths of nicotine, 2 mg and 4 mg. The manufacturers suggest that the gum should be chewed slowly and intermittently and its use should not be reduced until after about three months. I can see two dangers in doing this. Firstly, nicotine influences neuro-transmission, leading to induced states of arousal and relaxation by the effect of nicotine on nervous pathways in the reticular system of the brain. There can be no certainty that a patient will not become addicted to this new therapy. Secondly, there is a more sinister danger. There is a parallel in eastern culture – betel chewing and sucking (see below). Tobacco and other ingredients, wrapped in a betel leaf, are chewed slowly and intermittently over long periods.

Recent studies have shown that this is linked with cancer of the cheek which is more common in ethnic minority groups because of this popular Asian habit. There are two dimensions here: why use nicotine chewing gum when a cheaper substitute, 'betel', is available in Indian corner shops? and when we are trying to eradicate cancer of the cheek from betel addicts, what interest will it serve if we substitute smoking with nicotine chewing gum? Perhaps further research will throw more light on this hidden corner.

American sucking tobacco

Some American manufacturers want to market this product over here, although the DHSS has not been very keen to promote it[3]. This method is in fact no different from sucking the tobacco in betel. Again, why pay more to run the same risks?

Caucasians only

Glucose-6-phosphate dehydrogenase (G-6-PD) deficiency is usually more severe in Europeans than ethnic Afro-Caribbeans[4]. Favism has been observed only in Caucasians and is most common among Greeks, Italians and non-Ashkenazic Jews. It is an acute haemolytic anaemia, occuring after the ingestion of Fava beans *(Vicia faba)*, or broad beans, by susceptible persons with G-6-PD-deficient red cells. The anaemia may be very severe and accompanied by haemoglobinaemia. Beware of broad beans!

Ethnic Americans

Americans do everything in a big way and that includes drinking – even soft drinks[5]. It is not uncommon for a British GP to see an American patient with the symptoms of low-grade oesophagitis brought on by American dietary habits. This could be caused by reconstituted frozen orange juice, spiced tomato juice, black coffee or chocolate-flavoured milk and the symptoms can be burning, tightness, or pain in the chest, aching of the face or arms, or numbness.

ETHNIC AFRO-CARIBBEANS

Ackee

This fruit is a delicacy in Jamaica and is used in 'bush tea'. The ripe fruit can be eaten after a meal without ill-effects, but if it is unripe, it can be poisonous. It can cause hypoglycaemia due to two factors: hypoglycin A and hypoglycin B. This can result in vomiting (Jamaican Vomiting Sickness), coma and even death due to severe dehydration[6]. Three-quarters of West Indians living in the United Kingdom have come from Jamaica. They very often go home on holiday and bring back with them tinned ackee, which may contain unripe fruit. Indeed the US Food and Drug Administration banned the import of both fresh and canned ackee in March 1984.

Ethnic bilateral amblyopia
Recent evidence suggests that some healthy members of this group may suffer from bilateral amblyopia[7]. The cause is possibly genetic with or without some environmental trigger. The natural history is characterised by a short active phase terminating in an arrested phase. The features include a relatively rapid onset of bilateral failure of vision giving rise to reading difficulty, usually in a young ethnic West Indian, varying degrees of central and peripheral perimetric defects, and a pallor of the optic disc.

Although I have not come across a paper about this condition in ethnic Asians, I remember seeing some such cases during my training in Pakistan. Perhaps further research is needed.

Pancreatic diabetes
Cassava (manioc or tapioca) flour is the major source of carbohydrate in the Afro-Caribbean diet. Current research reveals that diabetes in people of West Indian origin may have a different pattern of disease from the rest of the UK population[8]. Most are non-insulin-dependent and the frequency of hyper-osmolar coma is higher than that of keto-acidosis. It is suggested that there is a link between cassava and pancreatic diabetes[9]. The diabetogenic agents in cassava are thought to be cyanide-containing glycosides, including linimarin, which are found mainly under the skin of the tuber and accumulate in areas where the root is bruised and allowed to stand before cooking. Malnourished individuals are more prone to this condition and malnutrition, though rare, still exists in the UK, especially in those adhering to cult diets.

ETHNIC IRANIANS

Teeth-grinding
The English believe that this is a psychological symptom but Iranians think otherwise[10]. They think that grinding of the teeth is a symptom of threadworm infestation. An ethnic Iranian father may bring his child to an English doctor with this problem, expecting to get a stool examination to diagnose helminthiasis, and will be very disappointed if this is not done. Mutual understanding is required. No one should take the other for granted.

Severe oesophagitis
The Iranian habit of drinking very hot coffee may lead to oesophageal lesions and should be born in mind with a patient of this ethnic group presenting with severe oesophagitis.

ETHNIC ASIANS

No clinical history should be complete without an enquiry into ethnic habits and diet. Smoking habits and betel chewing among the Asian population need to be taken into account.

Betel (pan) chewing

It is relevant here to reconsider the account given in Chapter 7.

This is a unique Asian habit – an after-dinner delicacy – enjoyed daily by one-tenth of the world's population[11]. Its ingredients have a great physiological value. After all, cultural habits were based on so-called scientific thinking when they originated. The betel leaf is a source of vitamin C. The betel nut is an astringent. Limestone paste (calcium hydroxide) is a rich source of calcium and stimulates salivation. Catechu is not only an astringent but also a source of iron. Rose hips contain vitamin C and have a pleasant taste. Turmeric is used for colouring and silver foil is thought to be an aphrodisiac. Every betel seller will ask the customer whether he would like betel with or without tobacco. Most of them will choose tobacco. A few may choose to try additional 'special ingredients' – which can be hard drugs such as cocaine, LSD, etc. (see Figure 1, Table 1).

During the process of mastication, a person chats with his friends and relatives, therefore inhaling the chewed tobacco. This is in fact a form of 'passive smoking' and is similar to the nicotine chewing gum recently introduced in the west. In excess, it could lead to carcinoma of the lung.

Recent studies have shown that oral cancers are more common in ethnic minority groups and carcinoma of the cheek is most common among

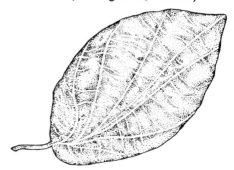

Figure 1 Betel leaf

Table 1 Betel (pan) chewing. A unique Asian habit. Used by one-tenth of world population. Side effects – cancer (cheek and lung) and stones (gall bladder, kidney, urinary bladder)

'The pan' contents	Reasons for use
1. Betel leaf	Carminative + vitamin C
2. Betel nut	Carminative + astringent (dries secretions)
3. Zarda (tobacco)	Nicotine – stimulant in small doses
4. Limestone paste	Calcium – to prevent osteomalacia
5. Katha (catechu)	Iron + astringent + protective against lime overaction
6. Cardamum	Carminative + pleasant odour
7. Turmeric root	Colouring
8. Silver foil	Aphrodisiac + nice presentation (in place of wine)
9. Rose hips (petal)	Vitamin C + pleasant odour

Note: Only adults use it and spitting is their social custom; chewed after food to deodorise the mouth; special receiver provided for its disposal.

the betel-chewing population[12]. There are two possibilities by which betel chewing can be responsible for this. Firstly, an unspecified amount of tobacco is kept against the inside of the cheek for long periods. This may affect the buccal mucosa directly. Secondly, limestone paste (calcium hydroxide), if not mixed sufficiently with water, has an abrasive action and can cause an ulcer which may become chronic and develop carcinogenic changes, resulting in cancer of the cheek.

The betel nut (areca) and catechu paste both have a strong astringent action on the buccal mucosa and are usually ingested, therefore affecting the intestinal mucosa. It is uncertain how these may affect the gall bladder, kidneys and the bladder but it is widely believed that these predispose to stone formation.

Biri

This is the equivalent of a cigarette and is widely smoked in India because it is very cheap. A specified amount of tobacco is wrapped in a biri leaf in the shape of a slim cone. It is never filter-tipped and towards the end the amount of tobacco increases due to the conical shape, and it is smoked to the 'bitter end'!

An English doctor is used to asking a direct question: "Do you smoke cigarettes?" An Asian patient may reply "No, Sir." Perhaps it would be better to ask if the patient smokes cigarettes or biri. In Indian cinemas and railway stations, the salesmen shout "Pan, Biri, Cigarettes!" Perhaps this should be the doctor's question.

Hooka

Smoking hooka, as mentioned in Chapter 7, is an Eastern habit. The hooka consists of a flask half-filled with water which is connected through a pipe to an earthenware funnel containing tobacco paste, covered with a stone disc, over which there are lighted coals; another pipe from the side of the flask above the water level is connected to a mouth-piece. As with the chestpiece of a stethoscope, this mouthpiece is never sterilised. One person inhales the smoke originating from the tobacco paste, filtered through the water, through the mouthpiece and then it is passed to the next person and so on among the family, relatives and visitors who sit around in a circle most evenings after dinner for a 'pow-wow'. This custom is not only popular in the Asian sub-continent but also is in vogue with the Arabs, Iranians, Chinese and south-east Asians. This was a sight very familiar

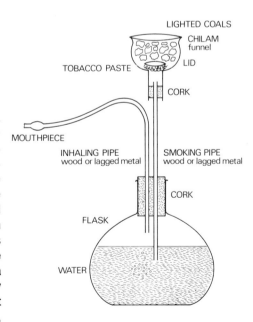

Figure 2 Hooka

to British Army personnel when visiting these areas (see Figure 2). There are many modified designs of the hooka.

This form of smoking is as dangerous as any other and should be elicited through direct questioning.

However, the Sikh religion forbids smoking and to a devout Sikh this would be an offensive question. Therefore an indirect approach is more tactful.

Pan-chewing is more common among Asian women and so they are more prone to cancer of the cheek and lithiasis. But biri is smoked by middle-aged Asian men who are then possibly more at risk of developing carcinoma of the lung. The hooka is enjoyed almost entirely by elderly men who develop a chronic cough which should not be taken lightly.

ETHNIC CHINESE

Cabbage and cancer
The highest incidence of oesophageal cancer in the world is in a remote valley in the Linxian county of China. This is attributed to 'Roussin's red ester', the presence of which is the result of a special preservation treatment applied locally to the cabbage[13].

Chinese cabbage is a delicacy and so may be imported from China. If a Chinese patient complains of oesophagitis it may not be attributable to hot drinks but should be investigated for the above possibility. This, of course, only relates to preserved cabbage from this region.

High salt syndrome
Analysis has proved that a typical Chinese takeaway meal has a very high salt content. Interestingly, the Chinese were the first to connect a high salt intake and high blood pressure: "If large amounts of salt are taken the pulse will stiffen or harden" (Huang Ti Nei Ching Su Wen; circa 200 BC).

Headache, thirst and a bloated feeling lasting up to four hours can develop after a Chinese meal.

Chinese restaurant syndrome
This controversial syndrome has been attributed to sodium monoglutamate, which is present in Vetsin – a Chinese food additive. In susceptible individuals the allergic reactions, lasting for up to an hour, may be thumping headache, burning, tightness or pain in the chest, neck, face or arms[14]. Some Chinese believe that it can cause alopecia.

Ginger Bezoars
Preserved ginger root is a popular Chinese snack and if not chewed properly, or eaten in a hurry, can cause small bowel obstruction at the ileocaecal junction[14]. The ginger root consists of cellulose, which is resistant to gastric juices, absorbs water and swells up during transit through the gut. An elderly Chinese patient or a child may be a victim, complaining of pain in the right iliac fossa. This must be considered in the different diagnoses of acute abdomen.

CONCLUSION

Ethnic differences are a respectable entity in science and should not be mistaken for inequalities. All patients expect the appropriate treatment and a GP should keep an open mind about the hidden corners of ethnic medical history. All health professionals need to be aware of such new information: it may prove vital to save lives.

REFERENCES

1. McLoughlin, J. *et al.* (1984). Hidden dangers of sliced bread. *Br. Med. J.,* **289**, 441
2. Fowler, G. (1984). Smoking cessation. *The Physician,* July 25 – 28
3. Palmer, J. (1984). A sucker for chew tobacco. *GP,* 3 August, 13
4. Young, L.E. (1971). Glucose-6-phosphate dehydrogenase (G-6-PD). In: *Cecil-Loeb Textbook of Medicine,* p.1490
5. Kenney, R.A. (1980). Chinese restaurant syndrome. *The Lancet,* 9 February, 311 – 312
6. Donaldson, D. (1984). Causes and mechanisms of hypoglycaemia. *Faculty News,* **4**, 5 – 6
7. Editorial (1981). Bilateral amblyopia and race. *Br. Med. J.,* **283**, 88
8. Nikolaides, K. *et al.* (1981). West Indian diabetic population of a large inner city diabetic clinic. *Br. Med. J.,* **283**, 1374 – 1375
9. Keen, H. The nature of the diabetes syndrome. *Medicine International,* **8**, 327
10. Qureshi, B.A. (1983). Transcultural medicine. *Pulse Reference Series,* **43**, 29 October, 26 – 35; 5 November, 35 – 44; 12 November,41 – 47 (see Chapter 7)
11. *Encyclopaedia Britannica.* Betel, p.1029
12. Burton-Bradley, B.G. (1979). Is betel chewing carcinogenic? *The Lancet,* 27 October, 903
13. Pulse of Medicine. (1981). Carcinogen from preservation of Chinese cabbage. *Pulse,* 5 December, 49
14. Smith, S.J. *et al.* (1982). A new or old Chinese restaurant syndrome. *Br. Med. J.,* **285**, 1205
15. Anon. (1984). Ginger Bezoars. *World Medicine,* **19**, 34

CHAPTER 14

MULTICULTURAL CUSTOMS ABOUT BIRTH, MARRIAGE, DEATH AND BEREAVEMENT

One can never say never or always in life because there is an exception to almost every rule. No doctor can expect to see patients from only one ethnic group all his or her life. Therefore, this chapter is aimed to outline briefly some transcultural information as a starting point in a cross-cultural medical consultation.

Broadly speaking, there are two main cultures, six major religions, four common persuasions, and four ethnicities in the world today (Table 1). However, there are many subcultures, religious sections, mixed persuasions and ethnicities. Moreover, acculturation results in new cultural entities. For example, in Britain there are three significant 'Westernised Eastern' groups: West Indians (Westernised Africans); East African Asians (Anglicised Asians); and Asian doctors (trained in British style medical schools). Although it is not possible totally to integrate or segregate, it is useful to understand each others' customs.

Table 1   The British Nation today

Cultures	Western, Eastern, Westernised Eastern
Religions	Hinduism, Buddhism, Sikhism, Judaism, Christianity, Islam Persuasions (liberalism, secularism, agnosticism, atheism)
Ethnicities	Caucasians (Europeans, Middle Easterners), Asiatic (Asians), Negroid (Africans, Caribbeans), Mongoloid (Chinese)

BIRTH

Safety rituals
Infant and maternal mortality was high before the invention of modern analgesia, antibiotics, and obstetric procedures. Necessity is the mother of invention and religious leaders played an active role in spiritual, psychological, and physical healing by means of herbal medicine and safety rituals. Although declining, this practice still exists.

Many devoutly religious women, from all six major religions, may use safety rituals during pregnancy, labour, and the puerperium so as to avoid the evil influence which is believed to cause an illness or accident. Similarly, their newborns are religiously protected.

These rituals include: the wearing of threads, charms, metallic symbols, or ornaments; giving food or money to the poor or sacrificing an animal's life (a lamb, goat or chicken); and holding thanksgiving ceremonies at home or at the place of worship. The religious ornaments may be worn on the neck, upper arm, wrists, abdomen, and ankle. Holy water, blessed by a religious leader, may be sprinkled on the mother and the baby as a safety ritual. A health professional who shows respect to these beliefs will ensure a good doctor – patient relationship.

Naming ceremonies

Christians may give an already chosen name to a child and baptise him or her later. A Jewish child will be given a name after a religious ceremony. Similarly, Muslims will name their child after an elder has said 'Aazan' (prayer call) in his or her ears followed by a ceremony to recite the holy Quran.

Devout Hindus, Sikhs and Buddhists – all believing in re-incarnation and astrology – may wait a few weeks because the name has to be chosen by elders or priests after consulting holy books and star signs to ensure good luck.

In Eastern society, a person's first name is the given name, middle name signifies the religion, and the last name denotes the family. Sometimes, a family title (e.g. Sheikh) precedes one's name and the father's name is also added on.

Head shaving

The shaving of the head of the baby in the first year of life is a ceremony popular among Muslims and Hindus. Occasionally, even an experienced barber may cause a superficial cut by mistake. This should not be misdiagnosed as physical child abuse. The ceremony is called 'aqyeeqa' by Muslims and 'moondan' by Hindus. Guests from other religions may be invited.

Circumcision

Male circumcision (pp. 38, 166) as already mentioned is universal among all Muslim and Jewish men. It is purely a religious act, establishing the covenant between God and the believers.

Male circumcision, for purely hygienic reasons, is widely practiced in the USA, Canada, Australia and New Zealand. Non-religious circumcision rates in these Christian countries in 1983 were 85%, 40%, 40% and 10%, respectively [1].

Birth certificates

One's date of birth is considered very important in the West but not so in the Eastern culture. It is not surprising that an English person will give his or her age precisely when giving a medical history but an Asian, African or Chinese patient may not be so sure.

In the colonial days before 1947, the birth, marriage, and death of colonial subjects were not registered. Therefore, if an ethnic minority patient tells his age to be 65, and the doctor were to suggest that he looks older, the patient will be happy to agree that he may be 70 years old. A doctor should be wary of this guesswork, in good faith, when diagnosing age-related illnesses.

MARRIAGE

Married names

In Western society, naming customs include: calling the first name as the Christian name, even if it is not a religious name; labelling the last name as surname and placing it first in telephone directories; including sometimes an ancestor's name as middle name which is usually not a religious name; using title (Dr, Mr) with surname and not with first name; and considering a woman's surname before marriage the maiden name and changing it to the husband's surname after marriage. These customs do not prevail in the East and the opposite is the norm.

Some professional women do not change their maiden names after marriage in the West. Names are not altered after marriage among Asians, Africans and Chinese people. In these cultures, it is frowned upon to marry outside their own tribe, caste, or what is called 'brotherhood' and even marriage between cousins is fairly common for various reasons including marriage stability and preventing divorce along with its effect on children. However, consanguineous marriages are now genetically challenged.

Marriage symbols

Wigs are worn by orthodox Jewesses after marriage. The hair is considered as part of a woman's beauty, and it should not be visible to the general population after a woman has entered marriage [2].

Hindu women wear a red powder called 'Sindoor' in the parting of the hair on the scalp after marriage. In the event of the death of her husband, the wife not only stops wearing 'Sindoor' but also breaks her bangles.

Wedding rings are worn in Europe by women after marriage. In England, the ring is worn on the 4th finger of the left hand but on the Continent it is worn on the right hand. Some European men also wear wedding rings.

If such a marriage symbol has to be removed during a medical examination the patient should be given an explanation or counselled. Removal of the symbol without warning is considered as bad luck or a death-wish to the husband, and this should be avoided.

Polygamy

Monogamy is universal throughout the world. Some sociologists claim that polygamy is human nature. Procreation is considered essential by all religions but more strongly by Muslims. Therefore, only Islam allows limited polygamy (up to four wives) for a man only in special circumstances such as if the first wife were to be infertile. Women survived longer than men and positive consideration of their financial and sexual care was another reason. In some Arab communities it is a status symbol but in other communities this custom is declining. In England, only the first wife of a Muslim is considered the legitimate one, whereas, in Pakistan, second marriage is only possible with the permission of the first wife. The law of the land must be obeyed.

Marriage certificates

Registration of a marriage with a Registrar is a recent trend. In the East, only religious leaders performed marriage ceremonies and kept records and this practice continued even after 1947 when the colonial era began to end. Some

Asian, African, or Arab couples may not have marriage certificates but would provide substitute documents, from the magistrates in their country of origin, for legal purposes.

DEATH AND BEREAVEMENT

Symbolic colours
Muslims and Jews choose to dress the dead body in a simple white shroud and this is to signify the equality of all persons in death. Christians usually select white but do not place specific preference on the colour of the shroud and a person can choose, before death, to be kept in a suit or wedding dress after death until burial or cremation. Generally, Muslims bury the dead body in a white shroud without a wooden coffin.

Hindus and Sikhs select a white shroud for an elderly male. Married women are dressed in new saris, in shades of pink and red, but widows are generally dressed in sombre clothes. Some items of jewellery are also left on the dead body.

Colours of mourning clothes vary with culture or religion: black is the customary colour in Britain and other European or Arab countries; white is traditionally chosen by Hindu, Sikh, Parsee, and Chinese mourners; greyish brown is the popular colour among Ethiopians and pale brown is preferred by Iranians; yellow is the customary colour for the blacks in the USA and people in many Far Eastern countries; and purple or violet has been used at the funerals of royalty and clergymen in many European countries.

Attending a funeral in a wrong colour can be as hurtful to the bereaved family as a Christian inadvertently sending a sympathy card bearing the symbol of the cross to a non-Christian family.

Symbolic hair
As a symbol of death in the family: Jewish men are forbidden to shave their beards and must observe strict mourning for seven days; Hindu men observe the ritual of not shaving until the 11th day; and traditionally, a Hindu or Japanese widow's head was shaved on the third day following the death of her husband and growing of hair was forbidden for the rest of her life but this tradition is changing with time.

Death rituals
As a general rule, a nurse in a hospital or hospice should remember to do three things: to record the patient's religion and ethnicity on admission; to contact the next of kin or relevant local religious leader, if the patient is dying, for last rituals; in case of death, to wear gloves to straighten the body without touching, by skin contact, if the deceased belongs to another religion and to be guided by the next of kin or religious guide on how to manage the dead body.

In addition to the six major religions and four persuasions there are many other religious sects – e.g. Jehovah's Witnesses, Mormons, Christian Scientists, Rastafarians, Bahais, Parsees, and so on. There are vast differences between the rituals among all these groups for the dying, management of the dead body, attitudes to post-mortems and organ donation, funeral preparations, and ways of consoling the bereaved relatives. Moreover, people are more sensitive at the time of grief, therefore it is helpful to read one latest book on this vast subject (see Further Reading), but a health professional should ultimately rely on being guided by the bereaved's next of kin and appropriate religious expert. Appendix 2 (p.225) summarizes customs regarding mourning and disposal of the body.

Bereavement approach

Kind words cost nothing but mean a lot. It will comfort the bereaved relatives immensely if a health professional were to say to a Christian or a Jewish relative that the deceased died peacefully; to a Muslim that the deceased appeared to say last words as 'Allah'; to a Hindu or a Sikh that the person died reciting 'Bhagwan'; and similar kind words for relatives from other religions.

Problems such as post-mortem examination, blood transfusion to the dying, donation of the body for research and teaching, organ transplants, abortion and stillbirth, and funerals should all be tactfully discussed with the bereaved's next of kin in each case. There are many differences in religious beliefs and cultural customs about these matters, but with tact most situations can be handled successfully. Finally, appropriate bereavement counselling should be provided where acceptable by the bereaved relatives.

CONCLUSION

Health professionals look after a patient from the cradle to the grave and beyond. Although I had enough information to write a new book on these four subjects I was only able to cover some practical issues because of the limitation on space in this chapter. Hopefully, this brief account should be sufficient to stimulate the reader to learn more in this newly researched area. Just a word of warning: new knowledge is luggage, and it is best to travel light!

REFERENCES

1. Wallerstein, E. (1983). Circumcision: ritual surgery or surgical ritual? *Medicine and Law*, **2**, 85–97
2. Kopelowitz, L. (1985). Jewish patients and the British general practitioner. In: Pereira-Gray, D.J., ed. *Medical Annual, 1985*, pp. 244–253

FURTHER READING

Green, J. and Green, M. (1992). *Dealing with Death: Practices and Procedures. Part 3. Religious, Ethnic and Cultural Aspects of Dying and Death*. London: Chapman and Hall, pp. 147–230

CHAPTER 15

TRANSCULTURAL FACTORS IN THE CONSULTATION: THE THREE GENERATIONS CONCEPT

"Measure what is measurable and make measurable what is not" (Galileo).

Transcultural medicine is a new challenge to science where new measurements are urgently needed. Migration is the result of the economical and technological interdependence of all countries. British doctors, who are used to treating patients of their own ethnic group, are taken by surprise by the variations of the clinical data presented by ethnic minority patients in the UK. To bridge this gap, this section proposes the three-generation concept in medical consultations. It should be noted that this concept is a revised version of 'the three-generation' concept proposed in Chapter 9 on the section on the Basic Concept of Transcultural Counselling and Management. In Western thinking 'the first generation' are those immigrants who were born abroad; 'the second generation' applying to their children, born in the UK. Therefore a revision was necessary. My revised hypothesis is given below.

Three generations

It is essential to compare an ethnic minority patient with an English or Scottish patient because a British doctor has a very clear concept of the latter. The 'all or none law' can be applied to English patients whose cultural, religious and biological data is the same from one generation to the next. But 'something for everyone' has to be the rule applied when dealing with ethnic minority patients whose three generations differ in many ways.

The three-generation concept based on age, for use during a medical consultation, is therefore proposed as follows:

1. The first generation A – retired elderly people – are the dependant relatives of a working migrant. They did not choose to come to the United Kingdom, but were happy to be supported by their sons who left home to seek work in this country. These people will have 70% characteristics of their native culture and 30% acceptability of English culture. They will feel homesick and apprehensive of the British GP.

This material has not previously been published.

The first generation B – working men and women – in fact migrated to the UK to seek work and they have 50% characteristics of their native culture and 50% adoption of English culture. They feel at home in England where their work is and often go back to their countries of origin on holiday. They are happy to see the British GP but bring medical conditions associated with both cultures.

2.   The second generation – young people under the age of 21 – were born in Britain or have received most of their schooling here. They have 70% characteristics of English culture but retain 30% characteristics of their grandparents' culture. They feel completely British and feel like aliens when visiting their 'grandparents' countries of origin. They may even feel hostile towards their own ancestral culture. They prefer to see a British doctor and will mostly present with western diseases.

3.   The third generation – children under the age of seven – are obviously school children, toddlers and infants, born in Britain and reared on an English diet. They are 95% British and may reject non-English food, and their mothers sometimes bring them to the British GP, complaining of their lack of appetite which, in fact, is a dislike of non-English food. However, these children will feel no hostility towards any culture but, as they get older, will be interested in visiting their ancestral counties, in the same way that Australians and Americans visit the UK and Ireland, with a map of their family trees.

It is inappropriate to measure all these generations with the same yardstick. Let us consider each generation in turn, in the light of the medical model.

The medical model

The basic medical model consists of history, examination, investigations, diagnosis and management. The Royal College of General Practitioners has suggested that medical problems are physical, psychological and social. I would add to this list 'communication', 'religious (moral)', 'cultural' and 'specific ethnic'.
    This model applies equally to all ethnic groups in the UK – majority (English, Scottish, Welsh) or minority (Irish, Polish, Italians, Greeks, Cypriots, Arabs, Asians, Afro-Caribbeans, Chinese, Vietnamese and so on).

THE FIRST GENERATION A

Reasons for consultation

An elderly ethnic minority patient visits the British GP on his family's insistence that he needs medical advice. A British doctor is patient-orientated and believes in a patient's personal privacy. As with all non-British people, this patient has a family-orientated concept and believes in shared privacy. To him, a patient is a member of a family which lives in a community. It is not uncommon for him to be accompanied by other members of his family who would expect the doctor to tell them everything about the patient, and expect to be present when he is examined. A GP should be very polite in asking them to leave the examination room, because otherwise they take it as a threat. In eastern cultures the illness of a patient is the crisis of the whole family and this is a form of social security system.

An English receptionist, used to seeing an English patient sitting quietly in the waiting-room with his nose buried in a newspaper, will be startled when an ethnic minority patient arrives with some members of his family just before the surgery closes. This happens for two different reasons. An ethnic Asian patient will avoid queueing in the surgery because he believes in a free-for-all, unlike the British, who are strongly queue-minded. An ethnic Arab patient, usually a Muslim, is very strict about alcohol avoidance and will be anxious not to sit close to an English patient who may have come straight from the pub. A Sikh will avoid sitting next to a smoker.

The GP should gently advise such patients to wait in the queue or make an appointment (something to which they are not accustomed) – advice which they will happily accept.

To this elderly ethnic minority patient, the cause of his illness is both physical and spiritual. He believes that the cure is in the hand of God, who says that he should consult a healer. He, in fact, is doing his duty.

History-taking

Culture-shock is a real entity. The British GP faces name-shock whereas the ethnic minority patient feels colour-shock. Both will be momentarily at a loss but hopefully still smiling at each other. They soon get over the strangeness.

A language barrier with a Polish, Cypriot, Asian or Chinese patient is a frequent occurrence. Sign language is of no help at this stage and should be avoided because signs can be easily misinterpreted in different cultures. For example, 'thumbs up' is an insulting sign to Belgians, Greeks and Asians. Additionally, an Asian patient may look at the doctor's Royal College tie depicting an owl, and be horrified as to him an owl is a foolish bird which sleeps during the daytime and even at night does not work, and it is a symbol of bad luck, something he does not need at this time of illness. This is the time to seek help from an interpreter, possibly a member of the family who luckily has come with the patient to the surgery.

Afro-Caribbean, Asian or Chinese patients, particularly women, will feel very threatened and insulted if a British GP looks them in the eye because in their cultures, lack of eye contact is a sign of respect. The British GP should realise that avoidance of eye contact is not a sign of shiftiness, conceit or rudeness in eastern cultures.

To avoid offence, it is safer to ask for a patient's first or given name, rather than Christian name, because they may not be Christians.

Laughing or joking with a patient of this generation is misunderstood as laughing at them, and should be avoided. They do not like English jokes, but do appreciate a pleasant manner and a smile.

It is wise not to ask to see such a patient's passport for identity purposes or to look for his date of birth. In his time there were no birth registers in India or other Commonwealth countries where these have only recently been introduced. Such an innocent enquiry from the GP may frighten the patient and seriously damage doctor – patient rapport.

Clinical examination

There are three important points to remember:

a) In eastern cultures a rectal examination is taboo. This is the punishment given to the chief of an enemy tribe when captured, and is the biggest disgrace and insult that can be inflicted. A rectal examination is a cardinal principle in geriatric medicine and an elderly western patient is used to this. If a Chinese, Asian, or African patient has to be examined rectally, he should be counselled beforehand and no mention whatsoever should be made of this to his relatives. Other taboos in these cultures include the use of pessaries, suppositories, enemas and inhalers, a visit from a social worker and a referral to a psychiatrist.

b) The extended family system and arranged marriage system are based on the principle "the less you know of others, the more you stick to one". In Jewish and Muslim religions, men are segregated from women, even at the time of prayer. It is a cultural issue rather than an act of sex discrimination for a male patient to ask for a male doctor, and a woman patient to ask for a female doctor. However, with tactful handling this point is negotiable.

c) Some religious symbols can appear frightening, but they are really innocent. For example, a Sikh may be wearing a kirpan (dagger) under his clothes. A HIndu Gujrati woman may have tattooes of swastikas on her forearms but she has no love for the Nazis or any quarrel with the Jews.

   Most elderly ethnic minority patients will take longer to undress for examination because, unlike their British counterparts, they are not used to swimming or sunbathing.

GP management

An English or Scottish patient likes to discuss his problems with his doctor and may be content with simple advice. An elderly ethnic minority patient wants a simple explanation rather than discussion, believes in drug therapy rather than counselling, and at the end of the consultation he expects a prescription, preferably for an injection because in his country of origin this is the only pure form of medication. He will compromise on tablets if given an explanation that they, too, are a pure medication.

He believes in *perhaiz*, avoidance of certain foods during an illness. He has been brought up with the idea that foods cause allergy and that during illness some food or other should always be avoided. The exclusion diet consists of three items – lamb, pears and spring water – because these are the foods least likely to give allergic symptoms. If a GP does not tell him to avoid a certain food relevant to his illness which he himself might suggest, he will turn to a Hakim or other alternative medicine practitioner who does believe in this theory.

Such a patient believes that certain foods are 'hot', e.g. meat, and other foods are 'cold', e.g. milk. He has the firm conviction that milk is harmful in colds and coughs and meat helps to cure them. This is probably based on the calorific value of foods, and some foods may influence the basal metabolic rate. Again, a good doctor – patient rapport can be maintained if each understands the other.

He will be delighted if the GP tells him to come for follow-up. He thinks that the GP is a family doctor who not only looks after his family but is also a member of his extended family system. If good rapport is achieved, he will be willing to negotiate or bargain on the GP's terms.

In the unlikely event of the breakdown of a doctor – patient relationship, such a patient will be polite and smiling, but very confused. He will tell the doctor what the latter wants to hear rather than the true facts, and get out of the situation only to turn to alternative medical practitioners or the friendly chemist.

Muslim patients will not accept alcohol-containing medications. In fact all Asian people call alcohol a *daroo*, meaning 'medicine', implying 'English medicine'. Near the time of death, devout Muslims refuse all English medicines, saying that they contain and smell of alcohol. A GP should reassure his Muslim patients actively that he will never prescribe any of the alcohol-containing medications, and that he is aware of the list (see Chapter 23).

It may sound a daunting task to deal with a first generation A ethnic minority patient because of lack of experience, but with patience, skill and tact a GP can soon learn to handle these patients and feel a sense of achievement as a result.

THE FIRST GENERATION B

The first generation B ethnic minority patients are the working migrants who will present with 50% of the problems of the first generation A and 50% of the problems of an English patient. In fact, they will put up with a 'generation conflict': the restrictive culture of their parents, their own compromising attitude with their workmates, and the free-style, anglicised attitude of their children. They will rebel against none of these, but this conflict causes them internal stress. They will feel angry if a GP patronises them. They will be over-sensitive about any gesture of denigration. Knowing that they had to migrate to this country and must make their venture a success, they will be co-operative at all levels. However, some may over-imitate and exaggerate either English or their native characteristics.

In addition, the following four points are worth mentioning:

Reason for consultation: If a patient is unhappy at his job and cannot get alternative work, he will face an avoidance/approach conflict. He may ask for a prolonged sickness certificate after an illness. At this point a GP can help him by making time to discuss his problems and enabling him to cope with them.

History taking: Most probably he can understand English, but his command of the language may not be satisfactory. He may misuse medical jargon which he has heard on television. If such a patient describes an illness in medical terminology, rather than a layman's language, the GP should tactfully go over the history again to get the true story.

Clinical examination: Although he will be embarrassed, he will agree to have a rectal examination, but would prefer this fact to be kept from his relatives.

Because of environmental stress, he may suffer from psychogenic impotence, but will be too shy to mention this to the GP. Instead, he may request a full medical examination. A GP should not take this request lightly and should ask why he wants such an examination. When the actual problem is revealed, the patient will need a physical examination of his genitalia and simple reassurance without this will not do.

GP management: This patient is likely to turn to alternative medicine and will not be able to afford a private consultation. He will be most grateful for a sympathetic GP's help.

SECOND GENERATION

These are the youngsters between the ages of seven and twenty-one, born in Britain. This is a special generation with new problems. They feel very British and present with English diseases except when returning from visits to their countries of origin. They speak with an English accent and will be very offended if a GP treats them as non-English and expects them to have non-English diseases. They feel very insecure because of a two-culture conflict – the strict discipline of their grandparents' culture and the freedom of their English peers at school and work.

In addition, they may bring the following four problems to the GP:

Reason for consultation: Some ethnic minority schoolgirls may deliberately become pregnant and even seek an abortion. This is a cry for help as a result of the stressful situation at home and at school, and may result in their having to leave both places. Should such a girl contact the GP, this is an occasion where he can make the best use of his primary care team.

History taking: There should be no language or comprehension problems. However, they may seek family planning advice in confidence and would not wish their parents to be informed, as these ethnic minority parents strongly disapprove of sex education and family planning advice for their children.

Clinical examination: In the case of an ethnic minority girl who has a boyfriend and may be using contraceptive methods, she is more likely to request a pregnancy test if her period is overdue for any reason. She may be terrified of becoming pregnant before marriage because such a happening will ruin her chances of an arranged marriage, even if she herself does not believe in this custom.

GP management: They will be extremely annoyed if a GP attempts to treat them in the same way as their first-generation grandparents, because some of them even feel hostile to their grandparents' culture. They may attribute their difficulties to their parents' culture and may blame the GP for not understanding their position. They expect to be treated in exactly the same way as their English peers. Nevertheless, their different genetic illnesses, based on differences in ethnicity, should not be overlooked.

THIRD GENERATION

These children under the age of seven are too young to have any cultural conflict as yet. However, the following four points may be noted in this group:

Reason for consultation: They may refuse to eat non-English food at home every day and as a silent protest may turn to chocolates and crisps. Their mothers may bring them to the GP, complaining that their children are not eating. In fact, they are not eating non-English food, but will happily accept English food, which they get at school.

History taking: An ethnic minority mother may have a problem herself, but instead of consulting the GP about herself, she makes the excuse that her child is ill. If, on examination the child is found to be well, the GP should not stop there, but ask the parents if they need help.

Clinical examination: Eczema and asthma are said to be more common in ethnic minority children born in the United Kingdom than those born in their countries of origin. Some studies attribute this to, among other factors, environmental pollution.

GP management: Some mothers will be over-protective, especially of a male child because in eastern cultures a male child becomes the breadwinner who supports the whole family financially. Grandmother is responsible for the care of her grandchildren, especially a grandson, because his existence ensures the social security of the entire family. Among Hindus, only a male child is entitled to set fire to the pile of wood for the cremation of a parent or grandparent.

CONCLUSION

A British GP will do well to follow these recommendations regarding clinical methods. It can be argued that he is not a leader – a leader only serves the interests of either the majority or the minority – but he is expected to be a provider of health care, looking after ethnic minority as well as majority patients.

MANAGEMENT OF ETHNIC ASIAN PATIENTS IN GENERAL PRACTICE

The media are giving increasing attention to Indian and Asian culture – and the British general practitioner is becoming increasingly aware of some of the physical, psychological and social problems that beset his Asian patients.

It is an unfortunate fact that to a British general practitioner all ethnic Asians tend to look alike. Nothing of course is further from the truth and it is time that general practitioners as well as other members of the community made an effort to distinguish between the different groups. Unless they have at least a basic understanding of their culture and characteristics they cannot hope to offer the help that is often so badly needed.

Broadly speaking, these patients come from four countries, four religions and four regions of the Asian subcontinent. The four countries are: India, Pakistan, Bangladesh and Sri Lanka. The four religions are: Hindu, Sikh, Muslim and Buddhist. The four regions are: North, South, East and West. It is of great clinical importance to appreciate the variations that exist not only in colour, height and weight but also in diet, customs and language (Table 1). Surprisingly, but helpful to the general practitioner, the common language is English.

ATTITUDES

Whereas English patients are familiar with the 'public schoolboy' demeanour of the British general practitioner ('hard' on the outside but 'soft' on the inside) and take it in their stride, ethnic Asians may react quite strongly to it, either favourably or unfavourably.

For example, elderly patients who served in World War II under Field Marshal Montgomery or Lord Mountbatten will appreciate the 'stiff-upper-lip' approach, whereas those who followed Gandhi with his 'non-violence but non-co-operation with the British' campaign may be put off by such a manner and follow their 'non-co-operation' reflex, in which case the doctor/patient rapport will be seriously damaged and result in non-compliance.

Another attitude that general practitioners should try to understand relates to the system of the extended family which operates in Asian communities. For example, the elderly expect to be fully employed until they die. A man will act as

First published in *The Medical Annual 1986*, ed. D.J. Pereira Gray, pp.155–165 (John Wright/Institute of Physics)

Table 1 Regional differences among ethnic Asians

Origin	Colour	Height	Weight	Food	Religion	Language
Pakistan						
Punjabis	Fair	Tall	Medium	Meat curry & chapati	Muslim	Urdu or Punjabi
Pathans	White	Tall and well built	Heavy	Tandoori meat & nan	Muslim	Pushtu or Persian
India						
Punjabis	Fair	Tall	Medium	Meat curry & chapati	Sikh or Hindu	Punjabi or Hindi
Gujaratis	Fair	Short	Light	Vegetarian or vegan	Hindu	Gujarati
Bengalis	Dark	Short	Light	Fish & rice	Hindu	Bengali
S.Indians	Dark	Short	Light	Fish & rice	Hindu or Christian	Tamil or Malayalam
Bangladesh						
Bangladeshis	Dark	Short	Light	Fish & rice	Muslim	Bengali
Sri Lanka						
Sri Lankans	Dark	Short	Light	Fish & rice & vegetable	Buddhist or Hindu	Sinhalese or Tamil
Kenyan or Ugandan Asians						
Punjabis	Fair	Tall	Medium	Meat and wheat	Hindu or Muslim	Punjabi or Hindi/Urdu
Gujaratis	Fair	Short	Light	Vegetarian or vegan	Hindu	Gujarati

a figurehead, security officer, wise man, family historian, arbitrator and, in some cases, commander. A woman may act as culture protector, folk remedial therapist, marriage counsellor, child minder, baby-sitter, chief cook, home help, night nurse, health visitor and family crisis adviser. In return they receive the 'financial' reward of food and accommodation, as well as the 'psychological' reward of being respected, wanted and loved. General practitioners who understand this will have a good rapport with such patients.

PRACTICAL PROBLEMS

Asian habits

Betel (pan) chewing. This is a unique Asian habit used by one tenth of the world's population to eliminate the smell of curry. It is done only by adults especially the elderly who have more time to spend on it than the younger working population. A special receptacle is provided for its disposal.

The 'pan', which is regarded as a delicacy, consists of a betel leaf, tobacco, limestone, betel nut, catechu and other ingredients. The tobacco and limestone may act as local irritants which may lead to a chronic ulcer inside the cheek which, if not dealt with in time, may become cancerous. An ethnic Asian patient who presents with an ulcer in the mouth should therefore, be examined carefully. A surgical opinion may be necessary before embarking on symptomatic treatment. Cancer of the lung is obviously also a risk and as betel nut and catechu are astringents, this could predispose to lithiasis – gall, renal or urinary bladder stones (see Chapter 13).

Spitting. As with the Greeks, spitting is a common Asian habit and in some areas there are council notices 'Spitting is prohibited'. Ethnic Asians may be more accustomed to using a handkerchief than tissues. This an important area for health education.

Hooka smoking. This is a shared social habit, very common among ethnic Asians, who sit around smoking tobacco through a hooka in a companionable way. A patient may deny smoking cigarettes, cigars or a 'biri' (Asian cigarette) but may demonstrate the symptoms of carcinoma of the lung. On direct questioning, he may admit to hooka smoking.

Karela. Karela (*Momordica charantia*) is an Indian vegetable and karela curry is becoming increasingly popular in the UK, not only among Asians but also the British, especially those who were in the British Army in India. Karela is a hypoglycaemic agent used by Hakims for treating diabetes mellitus, but it reacts with chlorpropamide to produce prolonged hypoglycaemia. An elderly ethnic Asian may come to morning surgery and complain of feeling very weak. Unless the causative agent is recognized, the condition could be mistaken for anaemia or depression. This diagnostic pitfall can be avoided by direct questioning.

Smallpox scars. Smallpox used to be quite common in the Asian subcontinent. Some elderly patients have smallpox scars, especially on their faces, which may be covered with hundreds of pitted scars. These scars may have caused deep-seated emotional problems in their youth because they would have been considered a great disadvantage in an arranged marriage. In old age, any inadvertent reference by the general practitioner could hurt the patient's feelings.

Religious issues

Hindu tattoos. A Gujarati Hindu woman may come to the surgery with various religious tattoos on her chest and arms. This may startle the general practitioner who is used to seeing tattoos only on sailors or workmen. Any derogatory comment by the doctor may offend such a woman, or her family. Some of these tattoos look exactly like a 'swastika', though it is in fact, the name of God – 'Om' – in Sanskrit. No Jewish doctor should feel alarmed. Some women and children go to India to have these tattoos ritually performed by specialized tattoo makers. Religious convictions run deep and should be respected.

Sikh kirpan. Everyone is now aware of the significance of the turban, but a general practitioner may be taken by surprise when he asks a Sikh to undress for examination and discovers the presence of an eight-inch curved, sheathed dagger under his clothing. By law, all guns and daggers have to be displayed in Asian countries, but in England all such arms should be worn under the clothing. The kirpan (dagger) is one of the five ritualistic possessions of a Sikh (the others being the turban, comb, special undergarments, and a steel bracelet). A general practitioner has only to stay calm and reassure his receptionist or nurse. Nevertheless this symbol should not be frowned upon or the patient will feel hurt.

Muslim purdah. Muslim women wear a veil in the presence of male strangers, including the doctor. This custom was introduced to guarantee the success of an arranged marriage. They may be apprehensive about being interviewed and examined by a male doctor and prefer to go to a lady doctor, especially for gynaecological examinations. Conversely Asian males are very embarrassed about being examined by a woman doctor. It is a traumatic experience which may require counselling. In Eastern religions this custom is not considered an act of sex discrimination − negative or positive − a compromise is needed.

Religious restrictions

Muslims. Pork, bacon, ham and lard, as well as alcohol, are forbidden. Any drug or food which contains these should not be suggested to Muslim patients unless it is life-saving, in which case counselling by the general practitioner or a Muslim priest will be required. There about sixty preparations prescribable under the NHS which contain alcohol.

Hindus. Beef is strongly prohibited. Some Hindus, especially Gujaratis, are vegetarians, and this should be taken into account. They will not accept vaccines prepared in egg or chick medium, such as measles, influenza and yellow fever.

Sikhs. Sikhs are not allowed to smoke or use alcohol. They are not even allowed to smoke the hooka, but they will chew betel which of course contains tobacco. They may be offended if asked directly 'Do you smoke?' An indirect method of questioning is recommended.

Cultural taboos

Rectal examination. This is considered a disgrace in the tribal customs of an Asian community. An ethnic Asian patient, especially a woman, will feel greatly humiliated if asked to undergo such an examination and will try to hide it from the rest of her family. However, in geriatric medicine a rectal examination is of cardinal importance. The doctor should therefore make time to counsel such a patient, especially if he wishes to demonstrate the case to trainees or medical students. Only in rare circumstances and even then with extreme tact should the fact that it is being done be revealed to the patient's family. This taboo also involves the use of enemas, suppositories and pessaries. Their compliance should be supervised.

'Low caste' parts. In Asian cultures the anus, genitalia and feet are considered inferior to the other parts of the body. The left hand is considered to be inferior to the right, and therefore this is the one used to touch or wash these three parts. A family planning nurse should be patient with an Asian woman who finds inserting a diaphragm difficult with her left hand. The doctor should handle such situations with tact and understanding.

Social services. In an Asian extended family system, the use of meals-on-wheels, old people's homes and referral to a psychiatric social worker are frowned upon. If such helpers are visiting an ethnic Asian's home, they should be very discreet and not tell inquisitive neighbours who they are, otherwise rumours might spread in the community which would denigrate the patient's relatives as being non-caring. Similarly health visitors, social workers and psychiatrists are taboo in Eastern cultures. A referral to a psychiatrist may jeopardize an arranged marriage.

Moral issues

The ethnic Asian will have strong views against euthanasia, abortion and family planning. Readers will recall that Mrs Gandhi lost her premiership when she pursued an enthusiastic family planning policy in India and was only re-elected after abandoning this policy. Where British patients will have views of rational morality, ethnic Asians will follow strict religious thinking.

CLINICAL PROBLEMS

Physical diseases

Holy water food poisoning. Some relatives who go back to India on holiday will bring back holy water or foods such as 'halva'. Owing to inadequate refrigeration and storage during transit, these may grow *S. typhimurium*. Traditionally the family will offer these holy gifts to relatives, who may become acutely ill as a result. Direct questioning and quick thinking by the general practitioner may be life-saving.

Malaria. Asians often go to visit their relatives in malaria-infected areas of the Asian subcontinent. A pyrexia of unknown origin in such a person should be investigated with this in mind.

Bovine tuberculosis. Some people who visit India like to drink fresh milk from a sacred cow. Such milk is not pasteurized and may contain tubercle bacilli. They may develop tuberculosis of the intestine, spine or glands, while their chest X-ray may be clear. Doctors should be aware of this common problem in order to avoid this diagnostic trap.

Amoebic dysentery. Hindus are very fond of building wells and *'Dharam salas'* (hostels for Hindu travellers on the lines of YMCA hostels). When on holiday in India, it is a sign of nostalgia to drink water from these wells, which are now very old and unsafe and may contain amoebae. The symptoms of amoebic dysentery may be mistaken for diverticulitis which in English patients is more often due to chronic constipation – a less common occurrence in an ethnic Asian patient because of his spicy food. It can also be mistaken as ulcerative colitis or spastic colon. Again, direct questioning and appropriate investigations are important. Steroids and surgery, commonly used for treating ulcerative colitis, can kill a patient with an amoebic dysentery.

Psychological illness

Impotence. The *Kama Sutra* is a popular book among Asians, but ironically the author was not popular in his lifetime. The author was a Hindu and the first sexologist in the world. Premarital sex is taboo in Asian society but sex within marriage is considered to be a duty. Anxiety, stress or responsibility relating to the extended family system may cause loss of libido in men, who may ask the doctor for an aphrodisiac before turning to alternative medicine. All that is required is supportive counselling.

Social matters

Family support. Many relatives may accompany an ethnic Asian patient to the doctor or visit when he or she is in hospital. The more the visitors, the more the respect and dignity of the person. An unwary receptionist or ward sister may feel angry and annoy the family by trying to restrict the number of visitors. A sympathetic approach is required.

Presents. English patients may give personal presents such as a thank-you card or a box of chocolates to the doctor or receptionist, but an ethnic Asian patient may choose to give them money. This can obviously be misunderstood by NHS staff, but it is intended simply as gesture of good will and not as a bribe.

Marriage between cousins. Although nowadays marriages between cousins are uncommon, they used to be very common because a marriage outside the family or the tribe was frowned upon. Therefore, surnames of the husband and wife used to be the same. Now some ethnic Asian patients who married outside the family may have different surnames because it is not customary to change the surname after marriage. Of course some English professional women retain their maiden names after marriage.

Communication difficulties

Culture shock. To an ethnic Asian who has been brought up in an Eastern culture, Western ways of life may cause culture shock. If such a patient is seen by an English doctor or nurse for the first time in his life, he may get a colour shock, and vice versa. This feeling will of course pass with time and should not be allowed to become a barrier.

Fear of prejudice. In Asian newspapers, the problems of religious conflicts and racial strifes are sensationalized and patients who like to read newspapers in their own language may need to be reassured by a Jewish or English doctor. English society is more tolerant of conflict, a fact which may not be known to an Asian patient.

Language barrier. Many patients may not be able to speak English because when they were young, it was the language of the rulers and they were discouraged from learning it. However, now they will be anxious to learn to speak English, if only a few words. The use of interpreters is an asset, and if health service interpreters are not available, a member of the family may help. As a last resort, help could be sought from voluntary organizations and religious institutions in the UK.

Prevention

Influenza vaccine. This is prepared in egg medium. Many Gujarati Hindus are vegans and will decline the offer of this vaccine. However, out of politeness they may not tell the doctor why they are refusing it. When a doctor considers that such vaccine is indicated for a chronic bronchitic, he may wish to counsel the patient. Such counselling can also improve compliance with measles immunization.

'Perhaiz'. This is a word used by alternative medicine practitioners such as Hakims. It means the avoidance of certain foods during an illness because many illnesses are considered to be due to food allergy. Some foods are considered 'hot' such as meat juice, and some are considered 'cold' such as orange juice. An ethnic Asian patient will ask his doctor about foods he should avoid. If he does not get an answer, he may lose faith in the doctor's treatment altogether, and turn to alternative medicine. The English concept of hot food being spicy or of high temperature is not, therefore, necessarily that of an ethnic Asian patient. To him, a food which exacerbates the symptoms of the common cold is 'cold' and that which improves the symptoms is 'hot'. When he has a cough, he may refuse to drink cold milk. I suspect a link in this concept with the energy value of foods and their effect on the basal metabolic rate.

Drug therapy

Insulins. These are of beef or pork origin. Beef is not accepted by Hindus and pork is forbidden to Muslims. If a patient is allergic to one and cannot have the other, he has a moral dilemma. The recent human insulin (synthetic insulin) is a misnomer, as it gives the impression of human flesh. Supportive counselling with the help of a priest or a community leader may help allay feelings of guilt suffered by a patient with strong beliefs who has to have insulin.

Alcohol. This is strongly forbidden to Muslims. Many medicaments which contain alcohol may offend their feelings. They may lose faith in the doctor who prescribes them and interpret such a prescription as a religious insult. Surgical spirit (70 per cent alcohol) given for an umbilical infection may anger a Muslim patient.

Acetylator status. Recent evidence suggests that ethnic Asians are slower metabolizers of drugs than the English. It may not be uncommon for an ethnic Asian patient to complain that he cannot tolerate the same dosage of antibiotics, antidepressants, antitubercular drugs or simple analgesics (he may say, 'I find it hot') as his English counterpart, and he may demonstrate side effects as a result. As a consequence, smaller doses of such preparations should be given.

Injection requests. An ethnic Asian patient may ask for an injection of pencillin rather than penicillin tablets for an acute infection. The reason is that in his home country, drugs in the form of tablets are not always given in pure forms and some preparations have been adulterated. As a consequence the patient has developed more faith in injections because these are usually refined and in a pure form. Simple reassurance that the tablets in this country are in a pure form and will be as effective as injections is all that is needed.

New problems

Doctor phobia. Many ethnic Asian mothers in the UK, admonish their children by saying repeatedly, 'If you do not behave, I shall take you to the doctor who will give you an injection'. This puts a fear of the doctor into him, only to be revealed in the surgery. 'Desensitization' is more appropriate than 'flooding' for this phobia.

Cultural anorexia. A diagnostic trap awaits the British general practitioner when an ethnic Asian mother or grandmother brings a male child, complaining that 'he does not eat well and needs a tonic'. If the child is normal, the doctor should resist the temptation to prescribe a tonic and use his skill in counselling or health education.

Counselling

It is essential for a general practitioner to understand differences in patterns of disease, compliance and response to drug treatment or medical procedures. Sometimes modifying the drug therapy or procedure may be sufficient, but on occasions supportive counselling may be required. A compromise has to be reached between what is required in the interests of the patient and what is accepted by that patient. When dealing with an ethnic Asian patient, the general practitioner should not hesitate to seek the help of local priests and voluntary organizations, who will be only too willing to help in addition to the primary care team.

CONCLUSION

By learning to understand his ethnic Asian patients the general practitioner will gain the trust of the whole extended family, and if he can employ a female doctor in his practice he will make it easier for ethnic Asian patients who want to retain their beliefs and ways of life.

CHAPTER 17

OBSTETRIC PROBLEMS IN MULTI-ETHNIC WOMEN

Transcultural medicine involves clinical and consultation encounters between a doctor of one ethnic group and a patient of another. European women are more likely to develop folic acid deficiency, due to lack of melanisation. Asian women are most likely to have osteomalacia because of their chapati diet and Chinese women have the highest risk of rubella. Ectopic pregnancy is most likely in Afro-Caribbean women due to their medically justified use of IUDs; thalassaemia, which is common amongst Cypriot women, is also found in some women from the Middle East, Far East and Asia. The appropriate use of iron, folic acid, vitamin D and calcium is essential. Cross-cultural differences are respectable entities and should not be taken as inequalities (see Chapter 11).

COMMUNICATION BARRIERS

Clear verbal and non-verbal communication is essential for good doctor – patient rapport.

Name shock

In an antenatal clinic, an interesting situation can arise. An English consultant obstetrician called Cholmondeley (pronounced Chumly) asks a Polish clinic nurse, Mrs Ocrimawicz ('cz' pronounced as 'ch') to call the next patient, a Muslim woman called Mrs Fakir, and to convey a message to the Sri-Lankan tea-lady, Mrs Wijayasinghe (pronounced V-J-sing-gay) to clear the empty cups. The nurse is reluctant to say these names out loud and turns to the Scottish registration clerk, Mrs Farquharson, for assistance. The resulting series of name shocks could easily end in confusion. As with colour shock, name shock is a real entity, adversely influencing rapport. This should be recognised and everyone should make an effort to pronounce each others' names in a convenient way.

First published in *Maternal and Child Health*, **10**(10), Oct. 1985, pp.303 – 307 (Barker Publications Ltd.)

Interpreters

As with first generation A (retired) women, first generation B (working age-group) women of ethnic minority groups such as Polish, Cypriot, Asian and Chinese appreciate the help of an interpreter, but second generation ethnic minority women, who most probably were born in Britain or educated here, are insulted at the suggestion that they have a language problem. This generation may instead have a two-culture conflict – the strict eastern culture of their parents and the flexible western culture of their peers.

Attitudes

A major survey by the West Midland Community Health Council revealed that some ethnic minority women dreaded seeing the maternity nurses because of their comments, such as "Why did you get pregnant again?" The patients felt that they were treated badly after delivery and one is quoted as saying "The nurse and doctor shouted at me and treated me like dirt". There may be various degrees of unspoken unintentional hostility, and a positive effort should be made to improve the situation.

In a Leicestershire study it was observed that Asian mothers had one and a half times the risk of perinatal mortality, when social class, parity, height, legitimacy and the GPs' qualifications of being on the obstetric list were taken into account[1]. If surveys were carried out among other ethnic minority groups, further needs would be identified. A lack of demand does not mean that the need does not exist.

RELIGIOUS MATTERS

An obstetrician is a provider of obstetric care for people from all denominations; he may himself be a religious person. Respect for the patient's religious beliefs strengthens the doctor–patient relationship.

Food taboos

There are six main religions in the world, Hinduism, Buddhism, Sikhism, Judaism, Christianity and Islam, all of which have food taboos and rituals. The obstetrician who remembers to ask the patient what is taboo in her religion will be rewarded by her full co-operation.

Latent diabetes

In patients with latent diabetes pregnancy may induce chemical or even clinical diabetes requiring insulin treatment. Insulin is available in only three forms, beef, pork and "human" insulin. Beef is taboo in the Hindu religion and pork is taboo in the Muslim religion, and these patients will not accept insulin from these sources. Although pork as a food is taboo in the Jewish religion, it is allowed in the form of injections, including pork insulin. Human insulin is a misnomer – it is, in fact, a synthetic insulin, though many devoutly religious people of different cultures think that it is made from human flesh (as described earlier on).

Time should be given to counselling patients prior to starting treatment with insulin, so that these aspects can be discussed. If a patient is allergic to all insulins except the one which is taboo in her religion, the obstetrician should contact the appropriate religious leader who will be happy to help and plead for the doctrine of the sanctity of life.

Hindus and Swastikas

Gujarati women are mainly Hindu and are vegetarians. They may have religious tattoos on their necks and forearms. One such tattoo looks like a swastika although it is, in fact, the name of God in the Hindi script. A Jewish obstetrician should not be alarmed when seeing such a woman in an antenatal clinic; certainly, no ill-feeling is intended.

CULTURAL ISSUES

Patient-orientation is an English concept. In the rest of Europe, Asia, Africa and South America, the doctors believe in the family concept. An English person believes in strict personal privacy, whereas in eastern sub-cultures, shared privacy is the norm. Some cultural habits give rise to medical problems.

Rubella risk

A Commons enquiry and a Charing Cross Hospital study revealed that rubella is more common in Chinese mothers than any other ethnic group[2]. One quarter of pregnant Asian women in the UK are susceptible to rubella; numbers of sero-negative Chinese, Indian and Pakistani women are higher. Women born outside the UK are nearly twice as likely to be sero-negative as those born within the UK probably because they immigrated after leaving school; rubella immunisation is not done in the countries from which they came. An obstetrician with multi-ethnic patients should bear this risk in mind.

Malaria reactivated

A pyrexia of unknown origin presenting in the antenatal period of a new immigrant requires early diagnosis and treatment because malaria can be reactivated by pregnancy.

The placenta is a privileged site where *P. falciparum* parasites may become sequestrated and develop into other forms. Such infected placentae have aggregates of reticuloendothelial cells in the intervillous spaces, areas of focal necrosis, thickening of the basement membranes and loss of syncytial microvilli. This is thought to retard intrauterine growth because of impairment of diffusion of oxygen and nutrients to the fetus[3].

Many Afro-Caribbean and Asian families visit their countries of origin on holidays. They are not accustomed to using malarial prophylaxis because they believe that treatment is only necessary after an illness has developed, but out of politeness they may not tell this to the doctor.

Chapatis and osteomalacia

The Asian population has the highest prevalence of osteomalacia of any group in the UK. Exposure to sunlight is equal in all ethnic groups in this country and clothing varies according to the climate. If the colour of the skin was the criteria for osteomalacia, fetal and childhood rickets, then ethnic Afro-Caribbeans would have a far higher incidence of these conditions than Asians, but this is not the case. Overclothing cannot be responsible for this because Asians are not all Muslims: some are Hindus and Sikhs and do not observe purdah. Indeed, many Muslim women do not observe purdah and go shopping in this country.

The explanation of this anomaly is a unique Asian dietary habit. Chapatis (Asian unleavened bread) are the staple diet of Asians only. This is their main source of carbohydrate and is eaten in large amounts daily. Chapati flour contains phytic acid which binds with calcium to make calcium phytate which is excreted thereby reducing the available calcium in the gut[4]. A function of vitamin D is to promote calcium absorption through the calcium-binding and transporting protein of the intestinal mucosa. This protein is not formed if there is vitamin D deficiency.

As a result of the daily chapati intake, insufficient calcium is absorbed despite the presence of adequate vitamin D. Thus both vitamin D and calcium should be given during pregnancy to prevent fetal rickets. To prevent osteomalacia which can result in a small pelvis, necessitating Caesarean section and the consequent risks, it is advisable that Asian children and adolescents, especially girls, should take vitamin D as well as calcium-containing foods.

ETHNIC DIFFERENCES

Certain genetic variations should be taken into consideration when dealing with multi-ethnic patients.

Melanisation and folic acid

The chief function of melanisation is the prevention of ultraviolet photolysis of folate and other light-sensitive nutrients. Studies have shown *in vitro* that human plasma loses 30 to 50 percent of folate in strong sunlight in one hour and *in vivo*, ultraviolet-light-treated patients show abnormally low folate levels (see Chapter 4). Therefore, in pregnancy folate supplementation is particularly necessary in light-skinned women. Ethnic origin should also be taken into account when interpreting haematological and biochemical tests.

Thalassaemia and iron

Beta-thalassaemia is prevalent in Cypriots, Greeks and Turks, and is also found in some patients from the Asian sub-continent and the Far East[5]. Iron tablets are strongly contraindicated in this disease, and ethnic minority pregnant women must be screened for haemoglobinopathies in antenatal clinics before iron tablets are given (Table 1).

Table 1   Ethnic distribution of haemoglobinopathies

Haemoglobinopathies	Ethnic distribution
Sickle cell disease	Afro-Caribbeans Mediterraneans Middle Easterners
Beta-thalassaemia	Mediterraneans Middle Easterners Far Easterners Indians Pakistanis
Hb C disease	Afro-Caribbeans
Hb D disease	Indians Pakistanis
Hb E disease	Far Easterners

Ectopic pregnancy

Ectopic pregnancy is the commonest cause of severe abdominal pain in ethnic West Indian women[6]. This is attributed in part to the fact that they often rely on intrauterine devices for contraception.

Multi-ethnic labour

In a London survey, significant differences were found in ethnic English, Afro-Caribbean and Asian women in obstetrical characteristics. Asian primiparae had the longest first and second stages of labour, with the highest incidence of prolonged latent phase and primary dysfunctional labour. Afro-Caribbean primiparae and multiparae had the highest incidence of secondary arrest in the first stage of labour and of primary dysfunctional labour, with the greatest recourse to emergency Caesarean section[7].

Asian women make a lot of noise during labour pains because culturally they are encouraged to express their feelings and not to bottle them up. This should not frighten the obstetrician or midwife, who may be only accustomed to English stoicism.

PRACTICAL POINTS

1. When doctor and patient come from different ethnic groups, in addition to the medical model (physical, psychological and social), it is essential to consider communication, religion, culture and ethnicity.
2. Iron must not be given routinely to ethnic minority antenatal patients until they have been screened for possible thalassaemia.
3. To prevent osteomalacia and fetal rickets in an ethnic Asian patient on a chapati diet, it is necessary to give not only vitamin D but also calcium supplementation.

REFERENCES

1. Clarke, M. and Clayton, D.G. (1983). Quality of obstetric care provided for Asian immigrants in Leicestershire. *Br. Med. J.*, **286**, 621–23
2. Anonymous. (1985). Chinese are words apart from GPs. *Doctor*, **15**, 3
3. Watkinson, M. and Rushton, D.I. (1983). Plasmodial pigmentation of placenta and outcome of pregnance in West African mothers. *Br. Med. J.*, **287**, 251–54
4. Campbell, E.J.M., Dickinson, C.J. and Slater, J.H.D. (eds.) (1974). *Clinical Physiology*, 4th Edn. Oxford: Blackwell Scientific Publications, pp.396–400
5. Wood, B. (ed.) (1974). *A Paediatric Vademecum*, 8th Edn. London: Lloyd-Luke, pp.115–117
6. Smith, A.M. (1980). Gynaecological problems in immigrants. *The Practitioner*, **224**, 913–16
7. Tuck, S.M., Cardoza, D., Studd, J.W.W., Gibb, D.M.F. and Cooper, D.J. (1983). Obstetric characteristics in different racial groups. *Br. J. Obstet. Gynaecol.*, **90**, 892–897

CHAPTER 18

FAMILY PLANNING AND CULTURE

INTRODUCTION

Transcultural medicine covers the clinical and consultation encounters which take place between a therapist of one ethnic group dealing with a patient of another ethnic group. It does not describe any one culture in detail, but covers all cultures, highlighting the interplay. This subject has to have a scientific basis and must avoid the realms of politics and emotion. In science, criticism is a positive activity.

This chapter is aimed at family planning doctors, including general practitioners, nurses, health visitors, pharmacists and administrators. My intention is to present ethnic, religious and cultural differences as a respectable concept because difference does not have to be considered as an inequality. I shall give a broad outline of clinical problems in dealing with patients from different ethnic groups, religions and cultures.

ETHNIC CONSIDERATIONS

Ethnic majority groups in the UK compromise the English, Scottish and Welsh, whereas ethnic minority groups include the Irish, Polish, Hungarians, Italians, Jews, Cypriots, Afro-Caribbeans, Asians and Chinese (see Chapter 2).

There are, of course, many variables, but let us examine four:

Retinal pigmentation

The retina is pink in Europeans but brown in Afro-Caribbeans, whereas it varies in colour in Chinese and Asians depending on the darkness of their skin. This point should be borne in mind when examining the retina of a patient with Pill hypertension.

Pill hypertension

Some ethnic groups have a genetic predisposition to hypertension, possibly due to increased salt intake and also hypersensitivity to salt. Recent studies have shown that Afro-Caribbeans fall into this category.

This material was first published in *J. Roy. Soc. Health*, **105**, No.1, Feb. 1985, pp.11–14 (Royal Society of Health)
Tables 2, 3 and 4 were first published in *Update*, **37**(5), Sept. 1, 1988, pp.406–410 (Update–Siebert Publications)

Drug response

Acetylator status is the rate at which the body inactivates a drug. There are slow and fast acetylators. According to one study, the indigenous population of the UK and the USA have 50% slow and 50% fast acetylators, but the Egyptians in this study were found to be 87% slow acetylators. Chinese, Asians and Afro-Caribbeans are therefore expected to be mainly slower acetylators than the English. A patient with slow acetylator status is likely to retain a drug longer, giving increased beneficial effects but also more prolonged side effects. Therefore, if an Afro-Caribbean patient complains that she cannot tolerate the Pill, she should not be accused of poor compliance, and an IUD inserted, without considering a lower dose Pill. Of course, this will apply to any drug (Table 1).

Table 1 Ethnic population and drug response (Studies with antibiotics, antidepressants and antituberculous drugs)

Clinical aspects	European population	Americans (white)	Eskimos (Canadian)	Arabs (Egyptians)	Africans (Ethiopans)	Asians (Hindus)	Chinese Japanese American Indians
Slow acetylators	50%	50%	5%	82%	83%	high percentage	uncomm
Fast acetylators	50%	50%	95%	18%	17%	low percentage	very common
Effect of a drug	average	average	less	more	more	more	less
Side effect of a drug	average	average	lower	higher	higher	higher	lower
If a patient cannot tolerate the recommended dosage for Europeans	stop	stop	stop	try lower dosage	try lower dosage	try lower dosage	stop

Notes: 1. A patient can either be a fast or a slow acetylator
2. Acetylator status means "the rate of inactivation of drugs by acetylation".
3. This clinical interpretation should logically apply to all drugs until statistically proved otherw

Melanin function

The chief function of melanisation is the prevention of ultraviolet photolysis of folates and other light-sensitive nutrients. An allowance should be made when reading biochemical results of blood tests on various ethnic patients. According to a Sri Lankan study, Pill-taking over one year led to lowered serum folates. i suggest in such studies, an examination of melanisation should also be taken into consideration.

RELIGIOUS CONSIDERATIONS

Contraception is a 'hot potato' in all religions. Even Governments do not agree on one policy; for example, the Pakistan Legislative Assembly pronounced that family planning cannot be an official policy of an Islamic country. Mrs Ghandi, who was the Hindu Prime Minister of the world's largest democracy, had to reverse her decision to back the family planning campaign officially in the face of public opinion. The Catholic stand on contraception differs vastly from the English policy. A family planning doctor, whether an English doctor treating a non-English patient or vice versa, must be very tactful if the intention is not to hurt the patient's feelings (Tables 2 and 3). Let us take two examples:

Muslim patients

Menstruation is a curse to a Muslim woman. She is not allowed to take part in daily prayers or Ramadan fasting during menstruation. If a doctor decides to insert an IUCD during this period in an Arab, Malay or Pakistani woman, he will need to explain, reassure and counsel this Muslim patient first. Although in keeping with the eastern concept of shared privacy one would discuss medical matters with the head of the family, i.e. the husband, this is one of the rare occasions when the husband would not like this to be discussed with him, because his wife would feel very embarrassed. 'Breakthrough bleeding' is considered as menstruation, and therefore causes problem.

Hindu doctors

Hindu women celebrate 'Brother's Day' and 'Husband's Day', whereas Christian women celebrate 'Mother's Day' and 'Father's Day'. On 'Husband's Day', a Hindu woman will pray for her husband's long life and should not be expected to give injections or insert IUCDs. Hindu women doctors very often ask for a day off on these occasions, and locum cover should be provided. Respect of a Hindu woman's feelings will result in increased co-operation.

TABOOS

Sex education

The arranged marriage system in the East is based on the concept that "The less you know of others, the more you stick to one". In the West, however, the right to choose is considered paramount, therefore, premarital relationships are based on the idea of "try before you buy". Eastern women, especially girls under the age of 16, would be offended if sex education was to be given as openly to them as to their western peers.

Table 2 *Family planning and religion*

Religions	Contraception	Procreation	Parents consent	Decision-making	Menstruation	Abortion	Sex Education
Protestant	Popular	Equivocal	Not essential	Personal	No taboo	Acceptable	Encouraged
Catholicism	Forbidden	Desired	Essential	Family	No Holy Communion	Strong taboo	Not welcome
Judaism	Frowned upon	Desired	Essential	Family	No sex during and 7 days after	Mild taboo	Not welcome
Islam	Frowned upon	Desired	Essential	Family	No sex and no fasting or prayers	Mild taboo	Not allowed
Hinduism	Frowned upon	Desired	Essential	Family	No prayers and no sex	Mild taboo	Not allowed
Sikhism	Frowned upon	Desired	Essential	Family	No prayers and no sex	Mild taboo	Not allowed
Buddhism	Accepted	Equivocal	Essential	Family	No taboo	Highly acceptable	Equivocal
Atheism	Popular	Equivocal	Not essential	Personal	No taboo	Acceptable	Encouraged

Table 3 Family and religions

Religions	Celibacy	Celibacy in marriage	Child marriage	Courtship	Unmarried mother	Common law marriage	Divorce	Homosexuality	Segregation of the sexes
Protestant	Frowned upon	Frowned upon	Not allowed	Yes	Acceptable	Acceptable	Allowed	Acceptable	No
Catholicism	Encouraged (e.g. monks and nuns)	Short term (rhythm)	Not allowed	Yes but no sex please	Frowned upon	Not acceptable	Not allowed	Taboo	No
Judaism	Not acceptable	Not acceptable	Not welcome	Yes but no sex please	Not allowed	Not acceptable	Allowed taboo	Strong	Yes
Islam	Not acceptable	Not acceptable	Allowed	Not allowed	Not allowed	Not acceptable	Allowed	Strong taboo	Yes
Hinduism	Not acceptable	Acceptable	Allowed	Not allowed	Not allowed	Not acceptable	Mild taboo	Strong taboo	Yes
Sikhism	Not acceptable	Not acceptable	Allowed	Not allowed	Not allowed	Not acceptable	Mild taboo	Strong taboo	Yes
Buddhism	Acceptable	Acceptable	Allowed	Not allowed	Frowned upon	Not acceptable	Not welcome	Not welcome	Yes
Atheism	Acceptable	Frowned upon	Not allowed	Yes	Acceptable	Acceptable	Allowed	Acceptable	No

Male doctors

A Muslim woman wears purdah and therefore all her life does not come into direct contact with any man except her husband. She is unused to being touched by any man, even a doctor during an examination. A refusal to be examined by a male doctor can be misunderstood by English health workers as an act of sex discrimination, but nothing is further from the truth, and wherever possible, a female doctor should be attached to family planning clinics, and if this is not possible, then a nurse should counsel the patient and a male doctor should reassure her and the family beforehand. Eastern women are shy for religious and cultural reasons and a nurse should remember that such patients will take longer to undress, and the receptionist should allow more time for such a patient, when making appointments.

Abortion

All religions favour the doctrine of the sanctity of life – all killing is wrong, whatever the circumstances. Although all religions will oppose abortion in principle, Catholics will feel far more strongly about this. In Japan (Buddhists) abortion is a contraceptive method of choice.

Pessaries

As with suppositories and enemas, the use of pessaries is taboo in Asian cultures. An ethnic Asian woman may show partial or complete non-compliance with the use of pessaries when given in conjunction with sheaths or in the treatment of monilial vaginitis. A health visitor can be extremely helpful in counselling and supervising such a patient.

Sterilisation

Male or female sterilisations are considered taboo in Indian and Chinese cultures because it is believed that afterwards their manliness or femininity is greatly eroded. Not only are counselling sessions needed before vasectomy or laparoscopic sterilisation, but also it is necessary to give post-sterilisation support.

Psychiatry

Psychiatry referral is considered taboo in eastern cultures, where arranged marriages are the custom and the extended family system prevails. Such a stigma may have far more damaging effects than an English doctor could imagine. If such a referral is necessary, it should be kept absolutely secret and the patient should be reassured of this privacy.

Domiciliary family planning

Chinese and Irish patients do not appreciate a home visit from a family planning doctor or nurse. They would much prefer to visit the clinic rather than risk their neighbours finding out because some of them may have very strong feelings against family planning.

VAGINAL EXAMINATION – REFUSAL

Asian

Asian women are reluctant to allow vaginal examination because premarital sex is considered such a great taboo that even after marriage, sexual inhibition strongly persists, and therefore, such an intimate examination, even by a family planning doctor, would be extremely embarrassing, although the patient may not say so out of politeness.

Chinese

Chinese women are normally of small build and the large vaginal speculum appropriate for European women would frighten them. A small speculum should be used routinely for Chinese patients.

Muslims

Because of purdah, these women will attend group practices where a woman doctor is on the staff. It is advisable to have two doctors consulting, one of whom should be female. Although all women hesitate to attend family planning clinics during menstruation, on occasions, such as for the insertion of IUCDs, this is necessary, and most will accept it. However, a Muslim woman will be extremely reluctant because of facing an 'approach/avoidance conflict'. These problems need careful handling.

CULTURAL ABORTIFACIENTS

An unwanted pregnancy has disastrous consequences for the social, economical and mental wellbeing of the parents – married or unmarried – the child, and society, who foots the bill. Abortion was considered as a method coping with this situation. In Japan, even nowadays abortion is one of the recognised methods of family planning. Due to conflict between the principles of religion and the practice of everyday philosophy, each country had to make laws, and in Britain the Abortion Act 1967 is such an example. In most cultures, openly or secretly, abortion is practised using various abortifacients and this may still be going on in England. A health worker might like to remember the following examples:

Western abortifacients

These have been sold in Europe for a century and were in use in Britain up to the 1960s. Their common constituents were aloes, apiol, tansy and ergot. In cases of threatened abortion, a gynaecologist should bear this possibility in mind and look for the signs or side-effects of any of these constituents.

English abortifacients

These were used even as recently as 1967, when the Abortion Act was passed:
Dr Reynolds' Lightening Pills
Silver-coated Quinine Pills
Menoroids
Pour les Dames (Moulin Rouge)
Occasional Capsules for Ladies
Quinine Sulphate
Ferrous Carbonate (Placebo)

American abortifacients

For nearly a century, the medical abortifacient used was Savin. The surgical method, still in use, is an injection of water into the uterus and then evacuation of the contents by a 50 ml syringe and cannula. A British gynaecologist should perhaps bear this in mind when dealing with threatened abortion in a patient arriving from the USA.

Malay – Chinese abortifacients

In Manila, after every Sunday Mass, a woman can buy an abortifacient remedy called 'Black San Miguel Beer' from a stall outside the church. When a woman buys the abortifacient, she is instructed to take it three times a day in memory of the Father, Son and Holy Ghost, and go on taking it for eleven days in memory of the eleven in the Rosary. She is told 'You drink it, there is pain and the bleeding begins'. What happens in Manila today happened in Birmingham in the 1960s and in Boston in 1900. One wonders if an ethnic Malay or Chinese patient can get it in England today?

SPECIFIC PROBLEMS

It is important for an English doctor to be aware of specific problems among ethnic minority patients. It is also essential for an overseas-trained doctor to understand the particular issues concerning ethnic majority patients. In a recent survey of multi-ethnic domiciliary family planning in Birmingham, the following situations were highlighted:

Ethnic majority

- *Large poor family* – in this survey, one woman was expecting her 22nd child; there was also a mother of eleven children. Some overseas-trained doctors are brought up to believe that the English family is always a nuclear family with two children.
- *Very young mother* – one girl had her first baby when she was fourteen, and a year later was expecting twins. I believe many school doctors and GPs are unaware of the possibility of pregnancy among schoolgirls.
- *Unmarried mother* – a woman who had had four children by four partners came to ask the doctor 'I have changed my chap, should I change my Pill?' My own feeling is that many Asian doctors will feel inhibited by their own cultural shyness when dealing with unmarried English and Afro-Caribbean mothers. A nurse can bridge this gap to the advantage of both parties.
- *Educationally sub-normal* – one such patient had had seven children, but was only able to look after one, therefore after each new birth, the older children had to go into care. I feel that a non-English doctor should familiarise himself with the social welfare system in England and pay a visit to a children's home.
- *Physically handicapped* – one couple (husband with multiple sclerosis and the wife with spina bifida) were no longer able to have intercourse, but asked the Family Planning nurse to continue visiting their home to 'save face' with their neighbours.

Ethnic minority

- *A West Indian woman* – in one instance the wedding could not take place because of the arrival of new babies. In another case, the partner refused to even consider male contraceptives.
- *An Asian family* – domiciliary FP is welcomed by Asian families. It is not uncommon to notice that if the nurse visits one patient, she could be asked to help another six neighbours. And, of course, there could be language problems, such as with the woman who said 'Husband no like – I like loop'. What she meant was that the husband would not have an IUCD for himself!

Dublin study

According to one study there is no official support for family planning in Ireland for religious, political, social and financial reasons. Therefore, family planning in Dublin is about fifty years out of date.

The Irish Law was very tactful, and said, before it was reviewed recently:
- Pharmacists are permitted to sell contraceptives but only on the production of an 'assessment' from a doctor.
- Doctors are permitted to give 'bona fide' FP advice. However, no-one was certain what is meant by 'assessment' or 'bona fide'.
- There were only two family planning clinics in Dublin. In 1981, it was observed that:

a) The attendance was growing
b) The Pill was the most popular method
c) IUCDs and caps were a social class variable
d) Two-thirds of the public health nurses opposed family planning
e) Domiciliary FP and vaginal examinations were not welcome
f) Guilt feelings among FP patients were a serious problem
g) Many patients went to their GP asking for the Pill to regulate their menstrual cycle
h) Many patients travelled from rural parts of the country to Dublin to seek FP advice. I suspect just as many travel to London for the sake of privacy, to obtain family planning advice.

METHOD PREFERENCE

It is impossible to make hard and fast rules about the most popular or unpopular methods in any one ethnic group (Tables 4 and 5). However, it is useful to have some idea of this. As a rule of thumb I would suggest the following:

Pill

This method is popular among the English who are well informed through the media on the pros and cons of the Pill and all its varieties. However, some ethnic minority groups with language difficulties may not feel confident enough to take the Pill. Here, assistance from a health visitor could be invaluable. Some Afro-Caribbean patients may not be able to tolerate the Pill if they happen to be slow acetylators, or prone to hypertension.

IUCD

Afro-Caribbean women find this a convenient method of contraception and there is no medication involved. However, an Asian patient will not like an IUCD because of the cultural apprehension of having a foreign body in her uterus.

Rhythm method

This is extremely popular among Catholics and is in fact, the only method openly allowed by their Church. Chinese and Asians, however, will not readily accept this method. If they are Hindus, Buddhists or Muslims, they will consider the rhythm method a Christian method.

Injection

This has only recently been allowed in the NHS. Asians are very fond of injections because in some villages in Asia, injections were the only pure form of medication available. I do not know of any ethnic group who would oppose it.

Table 4 *Contraceptive methods and culture*

Method	English Scottish Welsh	Irish Polish Italians	Greek Cypriots & Greeks	Chinese	Arabs	Asians	Afro-Caribbeans
Combined Pill	Readily acceptable	Reluctant but acceptable (especially as period regulator)	Acceptable	Reluctant if language problem	Reluctant if language problem	Reluctant if language problem	Accept if tolerated
Progestogen Pill (Mini-Pill)	Acceptable (no inhibition of ovulation)	Acceptable	Acceptable if break-through bleeding	Acceptable	Reluctant	Reluctant	Acceptable
Injectable contraceptives	Considered	Considered	Acceptable	Very acceptable	Readily acceptable	Very acceptable	Readily acceptable
IUD (coil)	Acceptable	Reluctant	Acceptable	Acceptable	Some reluctance	Very reluctant	Very acceptable
Diaphragm (Dutch cap)	Acceptable	Acceptable	Acceptable	Acceptable	Not acceptable (use of left hand)	Not acceptable (use of left hand)	Acceptable
Condom	Acceptable	Acceptable	Acceptable	Common	Common	Popular	Popular
Coitus interruptus	Not acceptable	Acceptable	Acceptable	Acceptable	Popular	Very popular	Acceptable
Natural method (rhythm)	Not acceptable	Very acceptable	Very acceptable	Acceptable	Not acceptable (Catholic method)	Not acceptable (Catholic method)	Readily acceptable
Sterilisation (male and female)	Acceptable with reluctance	Acceptable with reluctance	Acceptable	Not acceptable	Not acceptable	Not acceptable	Not acceptable

Post-coital contraception

This will be frowned upon by devout religious people. They believe it to be a form of abortion.

Abortion

As mentioned already, among the Japanese this is the most popular method, but this idea would, of course, horrify Catholics, as indeed would contraception itself.

Table 5 Family planning care and culture

Issues	English Scottish Welsh	Irish Polish Italians	Greek-Cypriots & Greeks	Chinese	Arabs	Asians	Afro-Caribbeans
Choice of doctor	Equal	Equal	Female only	Female only	Female	Female	Equal
Choice of language	English	English Polish Italian	Greek	Chinese	Arabic	Asian languages	`English or African
Husband's consent	Not essential	Required	Required	Essential	Essential	Essential	Not essential
Morbid jealousy (male doctor examining)	Non-existent	Slight	Very strong	Strong	Very strong	Strong	Slight
Domiciliary FP service	Acceptable	Not welcome	Not welcome	Not welcome	Not welcome	Very acceptable	Acceptable
Preference: FP Clinic or GP Surgery	Both	Clinic	Clinic	Both	Surgery	Surgery	Surgery
Vaginal Exam. (patient reaction)	Most willing	Accept quietly	Accept reluctantly	Accept reluctantly	Reluctant but quiet	Reluctant and noisy	Accept reluctantly

Diaphragm/cap

This method will be acceptable to most ethnic groups. However, some Asian women will reject this method just as they reject pessaries. They do not like vaginal examination or vaginal insertion because these are cultural taboos.

Sheath

This is the most widely-used method throughout the world. The irony is that this is the only reversible method for men, and they do not like it.

UNCONVENTIONAL METHODS

Folk-lore medicine is practised by some ethnic groups and perhaps we should consider the following two beliefs:

Breast-feeding

In eastern cultures, breast-feeding is considered a reliable method of contraception. Therefore, it is not uncommon to see an Indian woman breast-feeding her child, sometimes even up to the age of two years.

Leucorrhoea

Some Asian women believe that if they have a non-specific vaginal discharge, they cannot become pregnant. Such women will refrain from asking for treatment, and a GP noticing such a condition in the course of an examination will need to counsel such a patient. This is an important area for health education.

FAMILY PLANNING NEEDS

GP service

This is needed for patients from all religions, all ethnic groups and all cultures.

FP clinics

These will be needed by English patients who prefer to have a thorough examination and discussion in a specialist setting. However, an ethnic minority patient who believe in an explanation by the doctor rather than a discussion, and may have reservations about frequent vaginal examinations, may choose not to attend these clinics.

Female doctors

A Muslim patient would prefer to see a female doctor and this, of course, is not sex discrimination, but simply cultural shyness. Moreover, this will solve the problem of the under-employment of women doctors so bitterly contested by Women's Lib!

Interpreter

East Europeans, Chinese and Asian women may need an interpreter. Where this is not possible, they should be asked to bring another family member along with them to interpret.

Domiciliary family planning

Afro-Caribbean and Asian patients prefer domiciliary family planning. In this way they can have a long chat in relaxed surroundings with the Family Planning nurse or doctor and at the same time look after their children, thereby saving the expense of employing a babysitter.

CONCLUSION

Family planning is teamwork involving the doctor, nurse, health visitor, receptionist, administrator and the pharmacist. Patients come from various ethnic groups. No-one approves of inequality, but no-one should dislike the differences in cultural beliefs and ethnic needs. Different needs demand different answers. The purpose of this chapter has been to highlight these varying needs and attitudes. Inadvertent aggravation of many cultural conflicts can be avoided by keeping an open mind on transcultural understanding.

CULTURAL NEEDS IN BIRTH CONTROL

The planned family is a western concept based on the idea of a nuclear family, consisting of husband, wife and two children. Almost all Protestants believe in this idea. In the rest of the world, however, the idea of the extended family prevails – a family with unlimited relatives and an unrestricted number of children. Catholics, Jews, Muslims, Hindus and Buddhists favour this idea.

A British GP believes in the model of a patient and the community, whereas a non-British GP (in the UK and abroad) sees society as a family and the community.

Clearly, it should not be taken for granted that the whole world believes in family planning. However, the realities of life have forced everyone to accept this practical suggestion. Fortunately, modern family planning adopts scientific methods.

All religions are against premarital or extra-marital sex. Some religions go a little further. A Hindu is advised to observe partial abstinence from sex. He is given to believe that semen is the elixir of life. Recent studies have shown that 19-nortestosterone is an anabolic steroid used by athletes for the last twenty years. In India, wrestlers are advised to abstain from sex to preserve their muscular strength. Taking a bath after intercourse is compulsory for Muslim couples. This must create some problems in the winter months.

A British GP should be able to understand the reluctance exhibited by an Asian woman to undergo vaginal examination. During such an examination, an Asian woman may cover her face and make exaggerated groaning noises. The GP should not be put off by this cultural over-reaction.

For a British patient, menstruation is a fact of life, but for a Muslim woman it really is a curse. She is forbidden to take part in prayers, Ramadan fasting, and to visit tombs while menstruating. She will refuse to have a vaginal examination and an IUD insertion or use pessaries for treatment of a monilial vaginitis during

First published in *GP*, April 5 1985, p.33 (Medical Publications Ltd.)

this time. In other religions a similar attitude is taken to a varying degree. A GP should not only consider these points but also remember that breakthrough bleeding due to a combined Pill or the progestogen-only Pill can cause disruption in such a patient's daily life.

The incidence of intentional pregnancies and abortions among ethnic Asian schoolgirls has recently been reported. This is due to a two-culture conflict – a strict eastern culture at home and a flexible western lifestyle among her peers. Such a girl may find staying on at school unbearable. She may become pregnant or have an abortion to avoid school as well as the home situation. Although sex education for Asians girls is not approved of by their parents, a school nurse or a GP would do well to give family planning advice and be on the alert for such an occurrence.

A British patient prefers the Pill because she likes to use a method which is under her own control. She likes to discuss the merits and side-effects of the Pill with the GP, whereas an ethnic minority woman will be content with simple advice.

An Afro-Caribbean woman may be unable to tolerate the Pill because of her slow acetylator status and genetic hypersensitivity to sodium leading to hypertension. Hence, Pill hypertension is more common in this ethnic group.

Some Asian women may need an interpreter due to language difficulties. Occasionally the interpreter may tell the doctor what he wants to hear rather than the actual facts, and may also be over-protective towards the patient. But this is a rare occurrence. Cloasma due to the Pill (or pregnancy) is more common in ethnic Asian women.

Some Chinese women may not like the Pill and may use a Chinese remedy from an alternative medical practitioner. Most Chinese restaurants are family-run and some women may develop fungal infections of the skin due to excessive humidity in the kitchens. They may be prescribed griseofulvin for this, which has an interaction with the Pill, making it less safe.

Some foreign visitors may bring special problems. Foreign Pills can be substituted by their British equivalents. Portal cirrhosis is more common in India. Alcoholic cirrhosis is more common in Ireland. Liver disease is a contraindication to the Pill.

SOME CLINICAL POINTS

When introduced, the vaginal Pill will have an ethnic problem. As with psychiatric referrals and suppositories, pessaries are taboo to Asian and Chinese women. If given this method, they may even tell the GP what he wants to hear but in fact, have partial or non-compliance with this method.

The British have a patient-orientated concept whereas all ethnic minorities have a family-orientated model. A British patient decides for herself, whereas a non-English patient has to consult the family for a decision. A GP would do well to understand that confidentiality for a British patient is based on personal privacy, whereas for a non-British patient it is based on shared privacy. Therefore the Pill for minors is a controversial issue, which needs a compromise.

A British patient considers postcoital contraception to be just another form of the Pill or an IUD, but for patients from ethnic minorities, this is a form of abortion.

With the progestogen-only Pill, the only problem is due to more frequent breakthrough bleeding which is considered as menstruation by Muslims and other religions, including Jews.

A British doctor may prescribe pyridoxine for Pill depression and premenstrual tension, whereas an overseas-trained doctor may prefer to give vitamin B complex preparations.

In menorrhagia due to an IUD, a British doctor will be keen to prescribe Epsikapron but an overseas-trained doctor has more confidence in calcium preparations which are widely used in Asia for menorrhagia.

Depo-Provera injections have been widely used in Thailand for some years and Thai and Malay women will be delighted to see this available under the NHS. Asian women have more faith in injections than oral medication because in India or Pakistan, injections are the only pure form of medication available.

The IUD is the most popular method among Afro-Caribbean women. Some of them may not be able to tolerate the Pill because of proneness to Pill hypertension.

Hindu women (doctors and patients) celebrate 'husband's day' and on that particular day they will not give or receive injections and IUD insertions.

Some Asian women are frightened of the thought of a foreign body in their uterus and they will either not accept this method or come to the surgery with even minor twinges of pain. However, most of them may be multipara and a medium-sized IUD will be better tolerated than a smaller size which may cause intermittent bleeding.

Diaphragms and spermicides or pessaries are happily accepted by British women. Asian women consider a vaginal examination, insertion of pessaries or touching their own vagina for any reason, a taboo. Therefore partial or non-compliance with this method may result. If such a woman has to have this method, then a family planning nurse's supervision will be required.

The condom is the most widely-used method for men, and men do not like it. Chinese women are said to prefer men to wear condoms.

SHYNESS IS PART OF ASIAN CULTURE

An Asian woman trusts her man to use a condom but will be too shy to see it. Therefore, a doctor can never know whether a condom is being used. In Asian cultures, shyness is so important that a husband and wife never see each other's genitalia in their lifetimes.

An Asian woman will not like a doctor to talk about giving an anti-fungal cream for her husband to use. On such occasions the GP should see the husband personally.

British men, whether single or married, will happily accept vasectomy. However, Asian and African men have great reservations about this. They think that by vasectomy they will lose their manhood. They identify this with castration, which used to be the traditional punishment for the chief of an enemy tribe. Fortunately, there are vasectomy counselling clinics in the UK.

First male contraceptive

19-Nortestosterone is being considered as the first male contraceptive. It is given by injection weekly for 13 weeks and the azoospermia which results can last for a further 14 weeks after stopping the injections. However, it reduces testicular size by half. This may be acceptable to Europeans but will frighten the life out of Asian and Afro-Caribbean men.

Other considerations

British women accept sterilisation where this is indicated. Afro-Caribbean women are reluctant to accept this because they develop keloid scars at the site of the operation. Asian women think female sterilisation, as well as hysterectomy, represents a loss of their womanhood. In the past, in Asian and Muslim cultures, a second marriage was allowed if the first wife could not bear a child. This fear of childlessness still persists.

Catholics strongly oppose abortion, whereas this is the method of choice for contraception in Japan. The rhythm method is the only birth control allowed by the Catholic Church and for this reason Asian and Chinese women consider it a Christian method. Therefore, it is not popular among Hindus, Buddhists and Muslims.

Breast-feeding is an effective contraception method. If a woman breast-feeds six or more times a day and for at least one hour a day in total, it will prevent ovulation for more than 36 weeks after delivery.

The Irish and Chinese do not welcome a domiciliary family planning nurse visiting their house due to the fear of being seen by the neighbours. Afro-Caribbeans welcome such a service. If such a nurse visits an Asian household, the client may invite several other Asian women to see the nurse for family planning advice at the same time.

It is inappropriate to treat all women exactly the same because there are biological, religious and cultural differences between British and non-British patients. A GP or a family planning clinic doctor can serve the whole of British society – not just a section of it – by keeping an open mind and being aware of the above transcultural needs.

COMMENT . . .
on Transcultural Family Planning Consultations

Transcultural medicine

Transcultural medicine covers the clinical and consultation encounters which take place between a therapist of one ethnic group dealing with a patient of another ethnic group. It does not describe any one culture in detail, but covers all cultures, highlighting the interplay.

Ethnic English women – discussion

Unlike ethnic minority patients, ethnic English women are more aware of the topics of the day discussed on TV, radio and in the newspapers. They will have more confidence in taking the pill and will not hesitate to question the doctor about its side-effects and an overseas-trained doctor should not take this personally. An English patient likes to discuss an issue with her doctor, whereas an ethnic minority patient prefers a simple explanation rather than a long discussion.

Vaginal examination – refusal

All women have some reservations about this, but it is taboo in some cultures.
Ethnic Asian women are reluctant to allow this because premarital sex is considered such a great taboo that even after marriage sexual inhibition strongly persists and therefore such an intimate examination, even by a considerate female doctor, would be extremely embarrassing. Such a woman will start groaning even before she is touched and will flinch during the examination. However, this should not discourage the doctor. Counselling before examination is essential.
Ethnic Chinese, Malaysian, Bangladeshi and Gujarati women are normally of small stature and a large speculum will certainly frighten them. An appropriate speculum should be chosen.

Muslim women – no pessaries

To a Muslim woman, menstruation is a curse and this includes breakthrough bleeding. Ethnic Arab, Malay or Pakistani women will be extremely reluctant to have an IUD inserted during a period unless the appropriate counselling has been given, and they would not hear of inserting pessaries at this time, should they have monilial vaginitis.

First published in *Family Planning Today* (FPA & HEC), First quarter 1986, p.5 (Family Planning Information Service)

Jewish women – no lovemaking

Judaism requires that women should not have intercourse until seven days after the end of menstruation. It is unscientific to consider breakthrough bleeding as a method of indirect family planning. If such a woman has to take the progestogen-only pill, more attention should be given in regulating her periods.

Hindu women – no injection please

Hindu women celebrate 'Husband's Day' when they pray all day for his long life and refrain from giving or receiving injections on religious grounds. Such family planning women doctors will ask for the day off and their IUD and Depo-Provera injection clinics should have locum cover. Hindu women patients should be given another appointment for such procedures.

Ethnic Afro-Caribbean women – Pill hypertension

This ethnic group has a genetic predisposition to hypertension, possibly due to increased salt intake and also hypersensitivity to salt, and obviously will be more prone to Pill hypertension. They are slow acetylators of drugs; therefore they retain a drug longer, giving increased beneficial effects but also more prolonged side-effects . Therefore, if such a woman complains that she cannot tolerate the pill, she should not be accused of poor compliance and an IUD inserted without considering a lower-dose pill first.

Ethnic Irish women – guilt feelings

The ethnic Irish are well-known for their large demand for cycle regulator pills by women. Like the Chinese, Irish patients do not welcome domiciliary family planning visits. Respecting their religion, they will not ask for the pill directly, but would consider a suggestion from an English doctor to go on the pill, especially if he says it will regulate their menstrual cycles. A doctor should positively take the initiative to alleviate their guilt feelings.

Conclusion

There is more to transcultural family planning consultations than meets the eye and every doctor could make her or his own list of cross-cultural needs of her or his patients. An appropriate service will ensure compliance. It cannot be over-emphasised that one should keep an open mind when treating multi-ethnic patients, and be fair to all patients on the list – ethnic majority as well as minority.

CONTRACEPTIVE ADVICE: HOW THE ENGLISH DIFFER FROM THE AMERICANS

"The English have really everything in common with the Americans except of course, the language" (Oscar Wilde). I suggest that by 'language', Oscar Wilde implied 'attitudes'. There are two striking differences between the practice of medicine in the United States and in Britain: in the former, firstly there is a great emphasis on private medicine and secondly, there is a much higher incidence of litigation, whereas in Britain, on the NHS, the family planning service is absolutely free of charge, and litigation in this area is almost unknown.

I shall confine myself to the concensus of opinion agreed upon by the medical profession and the Family Planning Association in the United Kingdom, comparing it with current American thinking on contraceptive advice. While reviewing a recent British book by Pauncefort and an American article by Budolf *et al.*, I came across the diversity of opinions which can cause confusion for international readers. This article is an attempt to bridge the gap.

ORAL CONTRACEPTIVES

Absolute contraindications

British medical opinion agrees with the Americans on the following contra-indications: cancer or suspected cancer of the breast, ovary, uterus, vagina or cervix; coronary thrombosis; pulmonary embolism; deep vein thrombosis; angina pectoris; stroke; and unusual or unexplained vaginal bleeding. In addition, it is suggested by the British that late pituitary dysfunction and disorders of lipid metabolism should be included. However, unlike the USA, hypertension is not regarded as an absolute contraindication in the UK.

Relative contraindications

There are certain manageable conditions which can be regarded as temporary contraindications. These include obesity, heavy smoking, known or suspected pregnancy and impending operations.

Age is a complicated factor. Both countries agree that it is inadvisable to give the combined Pill over the age of 45 and indeed, over the age of 35 in smokers. In such cases the progestogen-only Pill is an acceptable alternative until the menopause, which is around the age of 51 years in the UK.

First published in *J. Roy. Soc. Health*, **106**(3), June 1986, pp.77–79 (Royal Society of Health)

Cautionary factors

We prescribe oral contraception with caution and carefully monitor patients who have the following risk factors: hypertension, chronic cardiovascular disease, varicose veins, smoking, history of jaundice, diabetes, migraine, epilepsy, otosclerosis, multiple sclerosis, porphyria (the Royal malady), gallstones, renal disease, asthma, obesity, previous ectopic pregnancy (women should not use the progestogen-only Pill), severe problems such as pre-eclampsia toxaemia in an earlier pregnancy.

Unlike the Americans, we do not consider mild sickle cell trait, fibroids and anorexia to be cautionary factors. British family doctors favour prescribing the combined Pill to patients with sickle cell anaemia, a disease common among Afro-Caribbeans. The Pill is said to have a beneficial effect on this condition.

When faced with these factors, a family planning doctor in the UK bases his judgement on the following considerations:

a)   is the risk of one unwanted pregnancy more than the risk of being on the Pill for one year?

b)   how many cautionary factors are present?

c)   the understanding and self-confidence of the patient

d)   how severe is the risk factor?

e)   the availability of medical facilities to deal with any complications that may arise, e.g. Pill hypertension.

Shared responsibility

A British general practitioner or a doctor running a family planning clinic would normally do all the family planning work on his or her own, and it is not exclusively the domain of consultant gynaecologists, as seems to be the case in America. For example, if a patient had amenorrhoea, the Pill would be prescribed by the doctor but secondary care will be undertaken by a consultant gynaecologist based at a nearby hospital. I remember a patient with mitral stenosis who was on the Pill for five years. As a rule, we do not prescribe the Pill to such a patient, but on this occasion we did so and shared her care with a consultant cardiologist, and fortunately there were no complications. A GP is considered a 'generalist' who knows about the whole patient and it is not uncommon for a specialist to seek a GP's advice.

Clinical practice

We agree on 75% of the routine adopted by the American doctors. On the first visit a detailed history (personal, family, medication, social, gynaecological) is taken by a family planning-trained nurse, who also checks the weight and blood pressure. The doctor, having checked the history, then performs a general and a vaginal examination, including a cervical smear. The doctor will then examine the breasts and teach the patient self-examination of the breasts to be done before each period. Following adequate discussion, the patient is given a three-month supply of an appropriate low-dosage Pill. Possible minor Pill side-effects are explained which can include nausea, vomiting, headaches, breast tension, weight gain, loss of libido, depression, proneness to monilial vaginitis, problems with contact lenses, chloasma and, in the case of the progestrogen-only Pill, irregular cycle and breakthrough bleeding. Generally these problems disappear after the first two or three cycles on the Pill. If they persist, we do change the Pill and try for another three months before changing the method. After the second visit, at three months, every patient is seen twice-yearly. On those visits the nurse and the doctor check for side-effects and check the weight and blood pressure. The breasts are checked on each follow-up visit by the doctor. A vaginal examination is carried out annually and a repeat cervical smear is taken every three years. However, this routine can be modified if any problems present.

We do not follow the American routine of checking thyroid function tests, gonococcal cultures, sickledex tests in ethnic Afro-Caribbeans or blood tests for anaemia. In Britain, iron deficiency anaemia is usually detected at school medical examinations. Some health authorities arrange sickledex tests for ethnic Afro-Caribbeans when they first visit a dentist. There are special clinics for venereal diseases where strict confidentiality is observed and the majority of the public is made aware of the existence of these clinics, which come under the National Health Service. Any medical condition such as thyroid disorder is fully investigated by the patient's GP or at a local hospital. All this treatment is free under the NHS.

American idea

The old American idea that a woman who had been taking an oral contraceptive for a year or so should stop for a few months so that Pill use would be cyclical, fortunately, was never followed by British general practitioners.

Pill amenorrhoea

A patient who becomes amenorrhoeic while taking the Pill is not regarded as lightly in the UK as she would be in America. She is closely monitored, not only by the family planning doctor but also by a consultant gynaecologist and in some circumstances other methods of contraception are proposed.

Missed Pill

According to current thinking in the United States, if a patient misses a Pill for one day it is not a matter of worry, but if she misses for two days, then barrier contraception is advised. We strongly disagree with this. A patient on the combined Pill who misses a dose for more than twelve hours, or a patient on progestogen-only Pill who misses a dose for more than three hours, is advised to use barrier methods in addition to completing the course on the Pill. We emphasise to the patient that taking two Pills together after having missed one is not safe.

Twins after the Pill

I was interested to read in the American medical press the curious statistical association with pregnancies that occur within the first three months after stopping the Pill and the increased incidence of twins, a phenomenon the Americans find hard to explain. I have not come across any documented evidence to support this in Britain and none of my colleagues are aware of this possibility.

Breast-feeding and contraception

In this country the progestogen-only Pill is advised during breast-feeding because the combined Pill suppresses lactation. The degree of suppression of the volume of milk may vary from patient to patient, even on the same Pill. As a consequence, the worry about adverse effects of the Pill on the baby does not occur.

Over age 35

The Americans put all the onus on the patient about the increased risks of the Pill at this age. We do not do this. We discuss with the patient of that age the possible risks, and consider the following four factors:

1) age 35+
2) hypertension
3) obesity
4) smoking

If there is one risk factor, the patient continues the Pill under close supervision. If more than two risk factors are present, we may advise against the Pill. It often happens that the woman will give up smoking and go on a diet, and hypertension, if present, can be controlled, so that the Pill can be continued until the menopause or until a problem arises. We find this a reasonable price to pay to prevent the unacceptable risk of an unwanted pregnancy. Under the welfare system in Britain, society and the patient share the responsibility of an unwanted baby.

Surgery and the Pill

We agree with the Americans in stopping the Pill four to six weeks before elective surgery to avoid post-operative thrombosis. We expect the patient to tell her dentist or a casualty medical officer in an emergency that she is taking the Pill.

ALTERNATIVE CONTRACEPTIVE METHODS

Depo-Provera

Medroxyprogesterone acetate (Depo-Provera) has not been given approval in the United States, despite its use world-wide. However, in Britain, after a lengthy debate, it has recently been approved for use under the National Health Service. In fact, some working women find it more convenient to have this long-acting injectable contraceptive. The dosage is 150 mg intra-muscularly every three months. I am surprised that the Food and Drug Administrative authority in the United States is taking so long to make up its mind.

Silastic levonorgestrel implants

This progestogen-only implant is not recommended under the National Health Service but I suspect some private practitioners may be using it. They like to keep up with American developments.

Sterilisation

The Americans seem to recommend sterilisation to women over the age of 30 or 40 liberally, but we have strong reservations about this and it is only recommended if all reversible methods of contraception have failed.

IUCD in nullipara

The American practice of not supplying an IUCD to a nulliparous woman because of the increased risk of subclinical salpingitis and subsequent infertility is not followed in Britain. We insert many modern IUCDs such as the Copper 7 in nulliparous women and the manufacturers have a thriving business. Insertion under aseptic conditions by a specially-trained doctor carries a negligible risk of pelvic infection. A patient is followed up regularly; a second visit after six weeks and subsequently every six months. Age is no barrier for the insertion of an IUCD in Britain and we do not agree with the American practice of not inserting an IUCD under the age of 26. The history-taking and management of a patient with an IUCD is as thorough as one with an oral contraceptive, therefore any complications are as closely monitored.

CONCLUSION

Since the 1960s the media has both praised and condemned the Pill. It has been particularly noteworthy because of the very serious risks that exist for a tiny minority of women. Much research has been done in this area and a woman can rest assured that any developments or published research are not likely to pass by her unnoticed. This applies to all Pill-users, whether in Britain or in the United States. Similarly, alternative methods of contraception are constantly under review. There is no doubt that, in the field of contraceptive advice, Britain and America lead the way and a closer liaison between the two medical professions is essential to reassure patients.

FURTHER READING

Budoff, P.W., Darney, P.D., Speroff, L. *et al.* (1985). Prescribing oral contraception in 1985. *Patient Care*, **19**, 16–55

Coles, R.E. (1983). Post-coital contraception. *Br. J. Sex. Med.*, August, 17–21

Ford, S.D. (1984). Resistance to vaginal examination. *World Medicine*, **19**, 7

Howard, G. (1976). Injectable contraception. *J. Maternal Child Health*, December, 10–15

Jordan, R. (1982). Family planning in Dublin. *Novum (Schering)*, November, 10,11

(1984). Pill reduces folate levels – Sri Lankan Study. *World Medicine*, Jan 7, **19**, 45

Pauncefort, Z. (1984). *Choices in Contraception*. London: Pan Books

Potts, M. (1977). Sociological aspects of sexual medicine. *Br. J. Sex. Med.*, Feb. 26–27

Rutledge, E. (1982). Domiciliary family planning in a multi-racial society. *Novum (Schering)*, Nov. 9,11

Smith, P.A. *et al.* (1983). Deaths associated with intrauterine contraceptive devices in the United Kingdom between 1973 and 1983. *Br. Med. J.*, **287**, 1537–1538

CHAPTER 19

PAEDIATRIC PROBLEMS IN VARIOUS ETHNIC GROUPS

A multicultural approach to paediatrics can help in the identification, quantification and management of the problems of multi-ethnic children. White ethnic groups are more likely to have cystic fibrosis, congenital dislocation of the hip or a strawberry mark. Jaundice may be underestimated or missed in ethnic Afro-Caribbeans who have a high incidence of glucose-6-PD deficiency. Chinese eyes should be looked at more carefully as squint may be missed. Cultural child abuse may be prevented by social education of the Asian fathers by health professionals. If the Royal Colleges can provide advice on the ethnic minority as well as majority, the British Government will not have to look elsewhere in her responsibility to serve the whole of the British nation.

EDUCATIONAL CHALLENGE

Science deals with objectivity and reason, whereas religion emphasises subjectivity and intuition. However, both teach that no-one, but no-one, should close his or her mind to continued learning.

Ethnic terminology

In every country there is a majority and a minority. Britain is no exception. Under international obligations, based on reciprocity, the welfare of the minorities is the Government's responsibility. The British Parliament passed the Race Relations Act (1968), which has been monitored by the Commission for Racial Equality since 1976, when it replaced the Race Relations Board (see Chapter 2).

The Commission recommends and the Registrar General uses the following ethnic terminology in the UK: 'ethnic majority' are English, Scottish and Welsh. 'Ethnic minority' includes Irish, Polish, Italians, Jews, Asians, Arabs, Chinese, Cypriots, Africans, West Indians and so on. The word 'ethnic' is added for those minority people who are resident in the UK. 'White ethnic groups' is recommended instead of caucasians and Europeans. 'Black ethnic groups' stands for Afro-Caribbeans.

First published in *Maternal and Child Health*, **12**(1), Jan. 1987, pp.15–20 (Barker Publications Ltd.)

The Commission disapproves of the terms: coloured, immigrant, reappearing/imported/alien disease and half-caste. This is to avoid the element of denigration.

Paediatricians will find it easier, when communicating with all ethnic groups, if they familiarise themselves with this terminology.

Multi-ethnic education

The Royal Colleges – medical and nursing – appear to follow the policy that all health professionals and patients in the UK are English or English-like, for example Scottish or Welsh, and if not, they ought to be. They have not recognised the needs of the ethnic minorities, therefore – in good faith – all the education, training and standards are confined to the ethnic majority.

The British Government's responsibility is to provide health care for the entire British nation. It consults the colleges for advice on the ethnic majority but turns to non-college advisory committees for advice on ethnic minorities[1]. The medical press is now moving tactfully in a multi-ethnic direction; the *British Medical Journal* has published a book – *The New Paediatrics* – based on articles by John Black (1985) on child health in ethnic minorities. The latest textbook for the DCH – *Child Health* – edited by David Harvey and Ilya Kovar (1985) is the first book to adopt a multi-ethnic approach. All children are tomorrow's taxpayers!

Politics is science dealing with reality. Moderates in all centres of excellence are increasingly holding study days on improving the health care of ethnic minority children and eventually a multi-ethnic education will evolve.

RELIGIOUS MATTERS

The English society stresses an individual's autonomy and personal privacy, whereas ethnic minorities press for parental responsibility and shared privacy. The first concept is based on a liberal Protestant view and the other is consistent with minority religions: Catholic, Jewish, Muslim, Hindu, Buddhist and Sikh. The 'all or none' law is totally inappropriate in child care and should be replaced by the policy of 'something for everyone'.

Customs

Paediatrics is the practice of family medicine and a paediatrician or GP will do well if he or she shows interest in the patient's religious customs. A Protestant or Catholic child will be christened or baptised. Asking for the Christian name may startle non-Christians, and it is wiser to ask for the child's first name.

A Jewish or Muslim boy has to be circumcised and if this could be done under the National Health Service, it would produce much goodwill.

Hindus believe in astrology and wait for a sign before choosing the first name, sometimes for several weeks, but usually they give a name to the child before the deadline of six weeks set by the Registrar of Births, Marriages and Deaths.

A Sikh boy may wear a turban and be reluctant to take it off. Persuasion and bargaining are more appropriate than using force with such children (Figure 1).

Buddhists claim to have no rituals or taboos and this should be explored in ethnic Chinese, Malay, Vietnamese and Sri Lankan children.

Faith healing

If a doctor shows his distaste for a patient's beliefs, he most probably will never be told that an Asian or Afro-Caribbean child is being treated with faith healing (Table 1).

It is common for a Muslim, Hindu or Sikh child to wear a charm to prevent accidents and diseases. A Catholic child will most probably wear a crucifix.

It does not pay to put people's backs up: with tact and understanding a confrontation can be avoided and a compromise reached to establish good doctor – patient rapport.

Table 1 Faith healing – children

Disease	Treatment	Country
Asthma	Tragus punch (ear piercing)	India Africa
Epilepsy	Ritually hanging the child upside down in a ditch	Jamaica
Insect bite	Breathing over the wound after reading lines from the Holy Koran	Pakistan Bangladesh
Prevention of accidents and disease	Charms and offerings	Asia Africa

CULTURAL ISSUES

Migration is almost always occupational. It is natural for ethnic minorities to feel threatened and cling to their own culture. There are many examples of contradictory practices in Eastern and Western cultures. A difference of understanding could lead to a lasting misunderstanding. A positive attitude is essential in multicultural paediatric health care.

Child-rearing habits

The grandmother plays the role of a health visitor in Asian culture and unless she approves of the advice from health professionals, compliance could be in doubt. She may even tell the daughter-in-law that the child, especially if a boy, is not thriving and the mother may bring a normal child to see the doctor, asking for a tonic or appetite stimulant. Careful counselling and health education are needed.

Culturally an Asian family is father-dominated and an Afro-Caribbean family is led by the mother, whereas an English family expects both parents to share equal responsibility. It is wise not to ignore an Asian father or African mother and the grandmother in a paediatric consultation.

In Eastern cultures a mother is confined to her home for 40 days following the birth of a child and the relatives are expected to look after her. After this time she has to pay return visits to all these relatives, keeping with the extended family system. She may be reluctant to attend child health clinics within six weeks and may not breast feed her baby due to inconvenience and embarrassment when making all these return visits to her relatives.

Child carrying habits vary in different ethnic groups; these should not be denigrated and their medical consequences should be borne in mind (Table 2).

Table 2 Baby-carrying customs

English	–	Pram or buggy
Asian	–	Hip
African	–	Chest sling (kangourou)
South Americans and American Indians	–	Back sling (papoose)
All	–	Arms

Note: Excessive practices can have physical, psychological and social consequences on the mother and the baby.

Cultural child abuse

Physical punishment of children was common in all cultures and is now decreasing because of the opportunities for early placement in playgroups and nurseries.

The English personality profile is vision, hearing and touch, but the reverse is the case in ethnic minorities. If an English child has done something wrong, the mother or father will remonstrate with him, whereas a father from an ethnic minority group may resort to beating the child. Where an English parent may smack the child's bottom, an Asian parent may slap his face. Even a shoe or a stick may be used.

Stealing is considered the worst behaviour in Eastern cultures, especially in a girl whose arranged marriage can be jeopardised. The father is responsible for shaping the child's behaviour. In England, such a father gets into trouble. If a bruise is seen on a child, the English health authorities may call a case conference, report him to the police and take him to court, and indeed, he could end up in prison. Nowadays a teenage girl may threaten her father with this eventuality, even in a case of simple family disagreement.

If a doctor, headmaster, priest or a police officer tells the father not to punish his child unreasonably, he will willingly accept this advice because he appreciates the feeling of sharing his responsibility with the authorities.

Campaigns of health education, counselling and supportive attitudes from health professionals are essential to alleviate distress.

ETHNIC DIFFERENCES

Patterns of disease vary in different ethnic groups and the causative factors could be genetic, nutritional or environmental. In this short chapter I will highlight some likely consultations in the UK.

Medical consultation

A strawberry mark is more common in the white ethnic group. It appears in the first month of life on the head, neck or trunk as a small telangiectatic area. It grows rapidly with the child in the first year of life, becoming a raised, red, lobulated tumour with capillaries visible over the surface. It disappears over the next five years[2]. An English or Polish mother will be very worried and need to be reassured. She may consult the GP, the community doctor, the consultant and possibly a private doctor. An ethnic majority parent likes to discuss things, whereas an ethnic minority mother is content with an explanation. Every paediatrician should spend some time in allaying her fears.

Hernias are common in ethnic Afro-Caribbean children but the 'supra-umbilical hernia' is the most common. It is shaped like an elephant's trunk with the unbilical scar on its anterior surface. It can be associated with 'cutis navel', another anomaly more common in African children[3]. Both anomalies result from divarication of the recti muscles and heal spontaneously within five years. Strapping may delay closure by preventing normal movement of the recti and by encouraging umbilical sepsis[4]. These should be left alone and on no account should an umbilical hernia belt be used because the protruding knob of the inner surface keeps the gap open. Strapping with a coin is the traditional therapy in various cultures, and this can result in intestinal obstruction. Old habits die hard. A doctor who spends more time in counselling an Afro-Caribbean mother can save a child's life.

Clinical traps

Tanner's growth charts, the only measurement available in the UK, do not apply to ethnic Chinese, Malay, Vietnamese, or indeed to Bangladeshi, Gujarati, South Indian and Sri-Lankan children (Table 3). Ironically, in those countries the American charts are used. These children will normally be small and of light weight, in keeping with their parents' stature.

Ethnically, Chinese children have wide epicanthic folds and a strabismus could be missed.

Mongolian spots are common in Asian and West Indian children and may mimic non-accidental injury[5].

Table 3 Ethnic compliance – children

Medical offer	English	Ethnic minority
Height & weight charts (Tanner)	Suitable	Unsuitable for – Chinese, Malay, Vietnamese, Bangladeshis, Gujaratis, South Indians and Sri Lankans
Drug metabolism and response	Equal – 50% of the English population are slow acetylators	Unequal – more slow acetylators, therefore a drug may be retained longer in the body, causing more response and side-effects
Measles vaccine (as with influenza and yellow fever, all made in egg medium)	Acceptable	Not acceptable to vegans (Hindu Gujaratis and English)
Insulin – pork beef human	OK	pork – Muslim taboo beef – Hindu taboo human – confusion in the name
Alcohol – oral local (e.g. surgical spirit)	Acceptable	Not acceptable. Strong Muslim taboo for oral as well as local medications
Suppositories, enemas and rectal examination	OK	Unacceptable (considered very dirty)

Dislocation of the hip is more common in Italians and its incidence in the UK is one in 1000 live births[6].

Cystic fibrosis occurs in one in 2000 live births among white ethnic groups and is less common in other ethnic groups[7].

Severe neonatal jaundice may be missed or underestimated in black infants who have a high incidence of glucose-6-PD deficiency[8].

Many children's lives could be saved and the stress on many families could be alleviated if a doctor dealing with children takes into account a patient's religion, culture and ethnicity in addition to the medical model (physical, psychological and social) without getting involved in the politics of integration and segregation. After all, the scientific variables include age, sex, social class, race, religion and region.

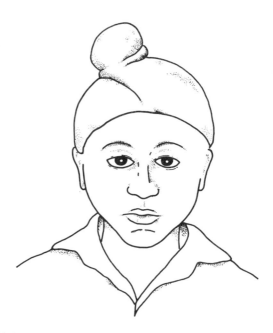

Figure 1 A Sikh boy wearing his ritual turban

PRACTICAL POINTS

1. Scientific variables include age, sex, social class, race, religion and region. A paediatrician can save lives if he takes into account the patient's culture, religion and ethnicity along with the medical model (physical, psychological and social).
2. An English parent may smack his naughty child's bottom, whereas an ethnic minority parent commonly slaps his face. The father could unwittingly exceed the limits of reasonable punishment. Social education of such parents by the health professional could save time, money and stress.
3. If in the past three years, you have not diagnosed any case of cystic fibrosis among the English, congenital dislocation of the hip among the Italians, non-pulmonary tuberculosis among the Asians, or jaundice in Afro-Caribbeans, do you think you could be wrong?

References

1. Citron, K.M. (1986). The future of BCG vaccination in schools of England and Wales. *Br. Med. J.,* **292**, 483–484
2. Verbov, J. and Morley, N. (1983). Developmental abnormalities. In: *Colour Atlas of Paediatric Dermatology,* Lancaster: MTP Press, p.16
3. Jolly, H. (1976). Congenital malformations. In: *Diseases of Children,* pp.273–275
4. Woods, G.E. (1953). Some observations on umbilical hernias in infants. *Arch. Dis. Child.,* **28**, 50

5. Black, J.A. (1986). Misdiagnosis of child abuse in ethnic minorities. *Midwife, HV Commun. Nurse,* **22,** 48–49
6. Harding Rains, A.J and Ritchie, H.D. (1975). Congenital diseases of bones and joints. In: *Bailey & Love's Short Practice of Surgery,* pp. 237–244
7. Dinwiddie, R. (1985). Respiratory diseases. In: *Child Health,* pp.185–195
8. Tarnow-Mordi, W. and Pickering, D. (1983). Missed jaundice in black infants: A hazard? *Br. Med. J.,* **286,** 463–464

Birth weight and feeding practices of infants in Southall, Middlesex

Asians represent a major group among ethnic minorities in the British community, and number approximately 800 000. In Southall, Middlesex, where 47% of the population are Asians, longitudinal data were collected over a 5-year period by one observer (BQ) on birth weights and feeding practices in a randomly selected sample of infants from four groups: Punjabi Indians, Pakistanis, East African Asians and English.

Female birth weights were similar to those for males in the three Asian groups. Birth weights for the male English babies tended to be higher than those of females but in both sexes were lower than national values (50th percentile 3500 g and 3400 g for males and females respectively; Tanner *et al.* 1966). Pakistani infants of both sexes were heavier at birth than Punjabi and East African Asians (Table 4).

Table 4 Birth weights (g) for infants by sex and ethnic group

Sex	English			Punjabi Indians			Pakistanis			East African Asians		
	n	Mean	SEM	n	Mean	SEM	n	Mean	SEM	n	Mean	SEM
Male	42	3445 *	70	75	3210	42	15	3300	82	8	3230	163
Female	44	3245	52	70	3175	43	16	3210	106	10	3075	96

Values exclude twins and infants with birth weights under 2500 g.
*Significantly greater compared with Punjabi male ($p < 0.005$); significantly greater compared with English female ($p < 0.01$).

The incidence of breast feeding for the whole population on which longitudinal data were available (124 infants) was 40.1%, and mean duration (9.5 weeks) was shorter than the national average (Wharton, 1982). By 26 weeks less than 2% of the population were breast feeding, the reason most commonly stated

First published in *Proceedings of Nutritional Society,* **42**(2), 1986, p.60A (Cambridge University Press)

(32%) by mothers for cessation of breast feeding was insufficient milk. Overweight mothers breast fed for a longer period (13.5 weeks) than either normal weight (7.7 weeks) or underweight mothers (10.7 weeks). By 12 weeks, 50% of all infants had received solid food, the most popular choice (80.0%) being commercial baby foods.

Tanner, J.M. Whitehouse, R.H. and Takaishi, M. (1966). *Arch. Dis. Child.,* **41**, 613 – 625
Wharton, B.A. (1982). *Arch. Dis. Child.,* **57**, 895 – 897

CHAPTER 20

PHARMACISTS' UNDERSTANDING OF CULTURAL CUSTOMS AND DANGERS OF MULTI-THERAPY

Medicine has two components: principles and practice. The principles are inflexible ideals and the practice is a compromise. It is desirable, yet impossible, for practice to coincide with principle. Sometimes there is contradiction. In such circumstances, the general practitioner has to make a difficult decision. As a rule, a doctor should prescribe what is appropriate for an illness; but in general practice, the patients' wishes considerably influence his decision.

Those wishes vary with personal, social and circumstantial needs. Instead of thinking rigidly in terms of right and wrong, a general practitioner or a pharmacist is forced to vary decisions in different situations. Making decisions aimed at solving specific problems is both desirable and possible. The patient is the most important person. His choice of therapies must be recognised. Medical principles disapprove of the use of the placebo, polypharmacy and 'multi-therapy'. In practice, however, these are widely used. Denying a problem does not help to solve it; but obviously recognising, evaluating and dealing with it is a step towards reaching the correct solution. Recently, an increase in prescription charges has reduced the patients' demand for both placebo and polypharmacy, but it has increased the use of over-the-counter medicine and alternative medicine. This results in multi-therapy, which has its hazards.

Let us examine three questions. Is there more to our patients than meets the eye? What sort of multi-therapy are our patients likely to use? Does it matter?

First, we are aware that normal drug activity differs, not only genetically, but also according to which ethnic group a patient belongs to. This can be measured by testing the acetylator status, (the rate at which a patient inactivates a drug by the acetylation process) in cases where it applies. Phenelzine, sulphonamides, and isoniazid are examples of drugs whose metabolism is found to differ in different races. The clinical response to drugs, including adverse side-effects will vary. Half the population of the United Kingdom and the United States are found to be slow metabolisers, compared with 1 per cent of Canadian Eskimos and 82 per cent of Egyptians.

According to a recent study, a patient with depression will improve more with phenelzine (MAOI) if he is a slow metaboliser, but will have more side-effects. We are aware of numerous drug interactions. The MAOIs, for instance, may cause a dangerous rise in blood pressure when interacting with tyramine-

This material first published in *Primary Health Care*, 1, No.4, March 1983, pp.9 – 10 (Newbourne Publications) containing foods like cheese, pickled herring, broad-bean pods, bovril, oxo, marmite, yeast and Chianti wine. Yet all these foods may be included in health food diets.

Tandoori nan (an Indian food) which contains yeast is becoming popular in Britain. Cough mixtures and decongestant nasal drops may contain sympatho-mimetic drugs. These may be bought over the counter. Their action, together with MAOI compounds, causes blood pressure to rise. This may lead to a throbbing headache, which is an early warning symptom. Further complications may follow. This example highlights drug – food interaction. It is the tip of an iceberg. The literature is full of such examples.

Secondly, we should be aware that many patients may receive treatment from the practitioners of alternative medicine, mainly for anxiety states, tension, chronic pain, allergies, psychosomatic disorders, chronic diseases and terminal illnesses. Patients will not go to them with acute illnesses or surgical conditions. Europeans may like health foods, herbal medicine and homeopathic remedies, whereas non-Europeans may visit a hakim (a herbalist and dietitian), an Ayurvedic practitioner (an elemental therapist), a faith healer, or may even undergo acupuncture or urino-therapy. Moreover, yoga and transcendental meditation may be practised daily.

Some dangerous drugs may be bought over the counter on holidays abroad. Patients may not necessarily tell their doctor about this; they tell him only what they think he wants to hear. Some patients, however, have communication difficulties with their doctors because of a social class barrier. They may conceal such facts in order to avoid annoying him.

Lastly, we examine the most important part of this discussion: does it matter? Take some common examples.

Homeopathic remedies: a patient with hay fever may use 'combination I' tablets (a homeopathic remedy). He may then come with ocular and nasal symptoms to his GP or pharmacist, who may prescribe eyedrops and a nasal spray. He will refuse to take antihistamine tablets, because of taking combination I tablets. The result will be partial compliance. One would never know which therapy was the successful one.

Health foods and medicine: a diabetic patient may be taking health food (medicine) with high vitamin C content (500 mg daily or more.) He may have a false negative result on urine test for glucose with Clinistix, when he may in fact have a profound glycosuria. This is because the enzyme in the Clinistix is inhibited by the ascorbic acid. As a result, the diabetes mellitus may remain uncontrolled.

Hakim's medicine: a hakim may prescribe a 'mercury kushta' (an aphrodisiac) to a patient over a long period. He may develop mercury psychosis (mad as a hatter), and may thus consult the GP, who may remain unaware of this fact despite having enquired about it. The GP may not then be in a position to manage the patient correctly.

Specific foods: drugs can also interact with specific foods used by different cultures. For example, according to studies reported in *The Lancet* and the *British Medical Journal*, an Indian vegetable, karela, potentiates chlorpropamide, which can induce a prolonged state of hypoglycaemia. Interestingly, hakims use karela powder to treat diabetes mellitus. Moreover, karela curry is becoming an increasingly popular dish in Britain.

Allergies

In addition, some foods may cause allergy. Practitioners of alternative medicine generally advise some form of dietary restriction. A non-European patient may startle a GP by asking which foods he must avoid.

Transcendental meditation and yoga: a patient receiving anti-hypertensive drugs who takes up transcendental meditation or yoga relaxation therapy may need a lower dosage. This relaxation therapy can potentiate the action of such drugs and cause hypotension.

The main difference between scientific medicine and alternative medicine is that the former is based on relaxing the body first with a drug, in the hope that homeostasis will follow. The latter involves relaxing the mind first, thus allowing the body to adjust itself. The advantages of non-drug approaches are that patients feel more relaxed, their high blood pressure can be reduced, and they get a feeling of euphoria. But there are disadvantages. Psychiatric patients may deteriorate and anxiety states may get worse. Symptomatic hypotension may develop. Meditation catatonia may occur. Even addiction to meditation may follow.

Drugs bought abroad: when on holiday abroad, a patient may buy 'Cibalgin' for relief of pain and in consequence suffer dental damage. Cibalgin tablets consist of allobarbitone 30 mg plus propyphenazone as a mild analgesic 220 mg, and insidious barbiturate dependency may result from regular use of them. The use of Enterovioform for travellers' diarrhoea may lead to paralysis of legs or optic atrophy. An infant may be given Lactogen (baby milk) and may develop 'bottle baby disease'. Such drugs are banned in Britain, but sold over the counter in third world countries. On returning to this country, a traveller may ask his doctor about side-effects, though conceal the name of the actual drug in order to avoid embarrassment. Remedies or other therapies which cause adverse side-effects may be purchased in the same way.

Prescribing

The result, as far as the GP or pharmacist is concerned, is that his patient presents problems of non-compliance or partial compliance. A drug given to a patient receiving multiple therapies could interact with or counteract with another remedy prescribed. The importance of this fact cannot be overemphasised.

What can GPs do about this? First, they should realise that patients may be resorting to multi-therapy but not be disclosing this for fear of disapproval. Second, GPs should positively ask their patients what other therapies they are using, taking care not to show a hint of disapproval in their question. In short, there should be better communication between GPs and their patients on the whole subject of multi-therapy.

The role of pharmacists as front-line health professionals is increasing and more patients are consulting them than ever before. The College of Pharmacy has put an academic seal on the quality of their training. The Royal Charter has been given to the Pharmaceutical Society of Great Britain. The pharmacists – in hospital or the community – should become ready to meet the new challenge of patients' increased expectations of them. High academic standards assisted by service with a smile will ensure the pharmacist – a member of the primary care team or not – a key role in patient care.

CHAPTER 21

MIDWIFE, HEALTH VISITOR AND NURSE: DEALING WITH PATIENTS FROM DIFFERENT CULTURES

Transcultural medicine comprises the medical encounters between a doctor or health worker of one ethnic group and a patient of another. It embraces the physical, psychological and social aspects of care and communication, as well as religious, ethnic and cultural issues.

ASPECTS OF CARING

Health visitor's attitude

A health visitor should be willing, without necessarily changing her personal views, to modify her professional approach according to the religious, ethnic and cultural needs of any patient from a different ethnic group. In return she will gain the confidence of the patient and ensure compliance with her advice. Patronising is a colonial approach, based on asserting one's 'superiority' on a patient with a different social background and ethnicity. Times have changed and this attitude is abhored by all ethnic groups. Then there is the 'Royal College' attitude. A public school-educated health visitor may believe, in common with some members of Royal Colleges, that all health workers and patients in the UK are English or English-like and if not, they ought to be. Ethnic minorities come from Commonwealth countries – black and white – and very much resent this approach. Ironically, our Royal Family have a much more humane attitude towards ethnic minority groups.

Health visitor's duties

Midwives, community nurses and even GPs sometimes have little idea of the role of a health visitor. In fact, she is a unique health worker who constantly supervises the growth, development and health of a child as soon as he or she leaves the security of the midwife's arms and right up until the age of five – school age.

First published in *Midwife, Health Visitor and Community Nurse*, **22**(12), Dec. 1986, pp.436–438 and 447 (Newbourne Publications)

Notification of Birth is done within 24 hours by the midwife who informs the District Health Authority, who in turn, allocates a health visitor to supervise this new baby – tomorrow's taxpayer.

The schedule of home visits is the eleventh day, three weeks, six weeks, three months, six months, nine months, one year and thereafter six-monthly until the age of five. GPs are well aware of the hazards of home visiting and should not underestimate the unique work of the health visitor, and should give positive support when needed. The health visitor sees the baby, mother and family. She advises on feeding, child care, personal hygiene, minor ailments, Social Security benefits and NHS facilities. A health visitor should spend sufficient time explaining these last two items to ethnic minority families who, unlike their English peers, may not be aware of these.

Home visiting

There are three basic concepts in home visiting.

1. *Extended family* – patient orientation is an English concept, popular among Protestants with liberal views. This gives rise to the nuclear family and patient-participation. All ethnic minorities – Catholics, Jews, Muslims, Hindus, Sikhs and Buddhists – believe in the family-orientation concept. The illness of such a person constitutes a crisis for the whole extended family, which includes grandparents, in-laws, relations and sometimes close friends. This gives rise to the term 'family doctor' and family participation.

2. *Shared privacy* – An English patient believes in the strict personal privacy so familiar to the English health visitor, and a non-English health visitor should bear this in mind. An ethnic minority patient exercises shared privacy, and the relatives expect to be present at consultations and believe that it is their right to be given details of the patient's illness because they then have to explain to other relatives what is happening to a member of their extended family.

3. *Religion* – ethnic minorities value their religion very highly. Religion is subjectivity and intuition whereas science is objectivity and reason. An English person may follow the scientific thinking which is: practical, analytical, rational and unemotional, whereas ethnic minorities follow religious behaviour: theoretical, empirical, moral and emotional. Whether a patient is English or from an ethnic minority, a health visitor (English or non-English) should tailor her approach accordingly. An Englishman's home is his castle, whereas an ethnic minority family hold an open house where anyone is always welcome to drop in and food is always available. A non-English health visitor should telephone first before visiting an English family, unless there is a special reason not to do so.

In Asian cultures there are superior and inferior parts of the body. The former include the face, right hand and right foot. The latter include the left hand and foot and the genitalia. It is considered bad luck if a health visitor enters a Hindu house with her left foot first. Hindus attach great importance to omens of good and bad luck. A left-handed health visitor should mention this at the outset to an eastern family. There used to be considerable prejudice against left-handedness in Asian society. Although decreasing, this discrimination still exists and is interpreted as a symbol of bad luck, and a visitor may be judged on whether he or she is a bringer of good or bad luck. An ethnic minority child showing a tendency towards left-handedness may be subjected to considerable cultural stress from his family, and this should be actively looked for because such a family will need tactful counselling and health education. Certain gestures signify bad luck. For example, if an English health visitor raises her hand to say hello to a Greek patient, to him it means a curse on his family. He will hide his face with both hands and may shut the door on her.

Interesting misunderstandings

An ethnic Italian health visitor called on a Vietnamese family (boat people) who were extremely polite but did not ask her to sit. As a result they all remained standing throughout the interview. In English culture, the host invites the guest to sit down. But in some eastern cultures the host waits for the guest to choose the best seat and only then will the host seat himself.

An English health visitor called on an Indian family who offered her tea or Coke. Her polite refusal was very hurtful to the hosts because in Asian culture a guest always accepts a drink or food. On another occasion, an Irish health visitor could not resist the repeated temptations of curry and chapatis when the hosts kept on offering them. In Asian cultures it is expected that a guest should know when to stop saying yes. An ethnic Kenyan health visitor decided to say 'I am fasting' when visiting, and this was accepted. Perhaps the answer is to accept in moderation.

After a home visit to a Polish family, a Chinese health visitor remained standing, chatting with the host, for half-an-hour in the hallway before they both realised that there was a cultural barrier; each was waiting for the other to open the door. In Polish culture it is the guest who opens the door on leaving, but in other cultures, the reverse is the case.

Clinic consultations

One of the major tasks a health visitor undertakes is to identify problem cases and arrange for them to see the GP, and then to follow them up. When dealing with a family of a different ethnic group, there are some cultural traps.

An English health visitor brought an English mother with a six-week-old baby to an Asian GP at his clinic for a check. The doctor found that the baby's head was not only large but the rate of increase in size was greater than the acceptable limits. The mother wanted to know everything about the matter and got very worried and upset. The doctor tried his best to reassure her that it could be a normally large head and that referral to a specialist, which he suggested, did not necessarily mean anything sinister. The mother then asked the health visitor, who tried to reassure her further, but told the GP "when she comes next week, tell her everything is normal". An English patient likes to be informed and to discuss the case with the doctor whereas an ethnic minority patient is happy with a simple explanation and reassurance. An English patient will be upset with the information if all is not well, but if a doctor tells her nothing is wrong when this not the case, she may end up sueing him. It is natural for a patient to be upset over bad news and a doctor continues trying to reassure her. This is a Catch-22 situation. An English health visitor should play a supportive role, helping both the mother and the doctor.

An Irish health visitor brought an Asian mother and her baby girl for a six-weeks check, complaining to the GP that she suspected child abuse because the girl looked "unhappy, Chinese-like", and although her height was at the 97th centile, her weight, which had been at the third centile, was now falling further, Failure to thrive is one of the recognised features of child abuse. The baby's older sister, aged three, also present, looked fit, happy and well-nourished.

On further questioning the mother told the doctor that she had had to stay at home for 40 days after the birth, as a cultural custom, but now she has to visit other relatives, especially for weddings, funerals and other ceremonies. She finds it very embarrassing to breast-feed the baby girl in front of other relatives but the health visitor insists on breast-feeding. She then asked the doctor if she could start bottle-feeding. The mother revealed that her in-laws are very sorry about the birth of the second girl because they are very old and this was the last chance for them to have a grandson, their eldest son's wife now being too old, after having two daughters, and the second son's wife being infertile. According to Hindu religious beliefs, it is the male descendant who lights the fire at the cremation ceremony. No wonder the child and the mother looked sad! Culturally Asians feed boys more than girls. Chinese waiters are rarely seen to smile – hence the health visitor's remark. A better cultural understanding is of great clinical importance in such a case and the appropriate feeding advice and counselling resolved the problem in this case.

Some specific problems

In Asian cultures the father heads the family. He is expected to keep a shoe or stick handy to frighten a child when, on his return from work, the mother tells him that the child has misbehaved. In fact, he makes a lot of noise hitting the floor or table rather than the child. It is similar to the technique of 'flooding' used by psychiatrists for shaping behaviour. This can be misinterpreted by English health visitors and social workers as child abuse. English mothers may smack a naughty child's legs, whereas an Asian mother will slap its face. All that is needed is to tell the Asian parents that this cultural custom should be modified in keeping with English laws. This advice will work like magic.

Giving the thumbs up sign and winking are common English habits. Thumbs up has a very rude meaning to Greeks, Asians and Belgians. It is akin to swearing. Winking by one woman at another woman is taken as an invitation to lesbianism, in Asian cultures. I suggest that an English health visitor should be very careful, when getting to know the mother from another culture, not to use such gestures.

An Indian mother believes that poor vision in a toddler is entirely due to too much television, and will expect the health visitor to support her in this and reinforce her warnings to the child. I am sure the health visitor would reassure her that there are a lot of good, educational programmes on television for children which they should watch, but they should not sit too close to the screen and should not stay up late. And, of course, the eyes must be checked in the clinic.

Although monilia on the tongue is common in all ethnic groups, lactose intolerance is more common among Asian infants. A health visitor is the most competent person to give advice on feeding, but in a case of suspected lactose intolerance, she should not start special expensive milks without consulting the doctor.

In some Asian cultures, especially Bangladeshis and Kashmiris, children are never given constructive toys such as building bricks, picture books, dolls' teasets or jigsaw puzzles. Therefore, they fail Stycar language tests and could be unwittingly recommended for special schooling. A health visitor should endeavour to persuade the mothers to buy English toys, and to let the children play with them all the time, rather than, as is the custom, only on special occasions.

An English educational psychologist believes lack of eye-to-eye contact is a sign of autism. This is not true in cases of Asian, Chinese and Afro-Caribbean children because, in their cultures, avoiding constant eye-to-eye contact is a sign of respect. A health visitor should avoid falling into this cultural trap.

And finally

The world has become a global village and, in keeping with other countries, the United Kingdom has ethnic minorities and for economic reasons it has to become a multi-cultural society.

It is a step forward for a health visitor to keep an open mind and collect her own transcultural information. She has nothing to lose. Her own work will be more enjoyable and she can save lives.

CHAPTER 22

CULTURAL ASPECTS OF THE MRCGP EXAMINATION

THE MRCGP EXAMINATION

The MRCGP examination is designed by the Royal College of General Practitioners on behalf of the British patient, conducted by a British examiner to test the knowledge, skill and attitudes of the British-born doctor who has been trained in a British medical school.

Similarly, in India a postgraduate examination is designed on behalf of the Indian patient, conducted by an Indian examiner to test the knowledge, skill and attitudes of the Indian-born doctor, trained in an Indian medical school.

This situation exists in every country in the world and **no** country conducts its national examinations as if they were organised by the United Nations. However, in spite of the fact that an examination is geared to the welfare of the ethnic majority of any one country, varying allowances are made for ethnic minority interests.

As with the English language and scientific knowledge, the MRCGP examination is a living thing. For example, since the point was made that the colour of the retina, with its diagnostic implications, varies in different ethnic groups, the examiners now show a slide of the retina of a West Indian patient, which is brown. And the examiners are now aware of the fact that the concept of 'don't know' is non-existent to overseas graduates – indeed, it invites punishment in some eastern cultures – and this column has been omitted from the MCQs, and 'yes', 'no' and 'don't know' have been replaced by 'true or false'.

The Royal Charter ensures the high standard of general practice and the MRCGP examination. It is in everyone's interest to reach that standard by further education.

The importance of cultural factors

There are many stories about the English in Ireland; however, one tale is very popular in Sweden. It is said that three Englishmen were shipwrecked on a desert island. Within half an hour of landing, they had formed three committees, each chaired by one. After one week they formed another committee to oversee the work of these three committees. It is natural for an English examiner to ask

This material has not previously been published.

questions about some Committees such as the LMC, FHSA, etc. An overseas graduate may lack experience of committees and may consider these questions irrelevant. He expects questions to be based on textbook knowledge.

In eastern cultures the concept of shared privacy exists due to the extended family system. One person's illness constitutes a crisis for the whole family. The GP is in fact a family doctor. Patient participation is exclusively an English concept. In Europe and the rest of the world, family participation prevails. To an Englishman, personal privacy is paramount, regardless of whether he is a patient or a doctor. It is not unusual, however, to visit the surgery of an overseas-trained doctor and see the receptionist sitting in the waiting room with all the patients' records visible, discussing each patient's symptoms in front of all the others. Asian patients thoroughly enjoy this, but an English patient would be extremely embarrassed. If such a GP presents his log diary to an English examiner and reveals all this, the examiner may encourage him to enlarge upon the role of his receptionist and will be very polite and not betray his inner feelings. And this well-read GP will never know why he failed!

One transcultural conflict can be laughed at. However, when there are ten such conflicts, it is no joke. Such transcultural encounters could be taking place in a doctor's surgery, an examination hall, at a job interview or place of work, resulting in communication breakdown. In this chapter I intend to highlight the cultural conflicts in the MRCGP examination without repeating the literature already available on examination methods.

Learning the correct attitudes

As with other postgraduate examinations, in the MRCGP examination three things are tested:
1. Factual knowledge
2. Examination skills
3. Desirable attitudes

A candidate may have a lot of factual knowledge and be an expert in examination skills but may have undesirable attitudes when dealing with a British patient or a colleague and therefore fail the examination. On the other hand he may possess the desirable attitudes and this may help the examiners to feel at ease with the candidate, so much so that any deficiency in the other two areas can be compensated for. There are excellent books and journals to update factual knowledge. In many courses the trainers go overboard in teaching the required examination skills. But there is no provision whatsoever for teaching the correct attitudes. The irony of this is that even the College says it has no official attitudes. This is a serious gap.

Attitudes are influenced by religion and culture. In England, one is free to practise one's religious and cultural attitudes but the English examiner, usually a Protestant, with liberal views, may not accept the candidate's attitudes. Due to the economic interdependency of the Commonwealth countries, there is a sizeable minority of doctors and patients who hold different views.

In the MRCGP examination where the attitudes desired to care for British patients are tested, it is clear that overseas graduates who have different religions and cultures suffer innocently (see Table 1).

Primary care involves more emphasis on attitudes than in other professional postgraduate examinations and this is obvious by comparing how overseas doctors fare in competition with UK graduates (see Table 2).

Table 1 Cultural comparison of pass rates in the MRCGP examination

Year	UK graduates	Overseas graduates
1980	60%	6%
1981	64%	5%
1982	70%	18%
1983	70%	25%
1984	74%	17%

Note:
1. Overseas trainees fared better than overseas principals. However, the opposite applied to UK graduates.
2. The rise in pass percentages of overseas graduates in 1982–84 reflected the mutual transcultural understanding at the Annual MRCGP Study Day for Overseas Graduates, held at the College, taught by 10% of the current examiners. The cultural attitudes, showing the differences, were identified by using the examination methods.

Table 2 Cultural comparison of pass rates in Royal College examinations (1980)

Examination	UK graduates	Overseas graduates
MRCP	42%	20%
FRCS	45%	25%
MRCOG	65%	35%
MRCPsych	69%	39%
MRCGP	60%	6%

SOURCE: John Fry, 1982 RCGP Members' Reference Book, p. 208

PREPARATION

Self-discipline

This examination is like a game such as cricket, in which the batsman faces a bowler and tries to score. A candidate in the MRCGP examination is invited to bat while a team of examiners throw questions at him to test his abilities, and he can only score if he has spent a lot of time and effort in preparation for the test. A person who lacks practice will be out as if it was 'LBW'.

A candidate needs three things: time, money and determination. On average one needs to study for eighteen months, at least four hours a day. Money is needed for books, courses and examination fees (and resitting!).

I have observed that an English candidate is honest with himself and if he cannot provide these three things, he will not attempt the examination. On the other hand, an overseas graduate practising in Britain probably has a non-working wife looking after a young family, making very justifiable demands on his time and money. A female overseas graduate most probably will be responsible for her family, husband and full-time practice, leaving no time for study.

I suggest that an overseas graduate be honest with himself and get his priorities right. An immature attempt at the examination, even if it is for employment reasons, wastes everybody's time and increases the failure rate.

Compensate for basic training

While giving talks on transcultural encounters in the MRCGP and FRCS (Lond.) examinations at both Colleges, I gathered from talking to the candidates and the examiners that they were too polite to be honest with each other. But they have genuine complaints (see Tables 3 and 4). I can appreciate both sides of the problem and strongly believe that if both parties are made aware of the truth, this gap could be bridged without either side losing face.

Table 3 Problems in transcultural examination encounters

"Overseas graduates do their best in all Royal College Examinations – yet their pass rates remain unacceptably low."

Overseas graduates complain
1. "I know it all – why do I still fail?"
2. "The examiner is colour-prejudiced."

English examiners complain
1. "The overseas basic training is different."
2. "They speak good English but a different language."

Table 4 Possible solutions

---

1. Lower exam standard
2. Alternative assessment – separate for overseas graduates
3. Forget it!
4. Further education

Overseas graduates qualify from British-style medical schools, reading books by western authors, but the teachers – who have a major influence in training – for nationalistic reasons are non-British. Moreover the patients are also non-British.

As English training is not quite right for those countries, so overseas training is inappropriate for British general practice. Such candidates, contrary to common belief, fail the papers as well as the orals, showing that the medical school training for basic qualifications varies from one country to another. Perhaps an overseas graduate should read the textbooks used by final year medical students in British medical schools and when preparing for this examination, should visit a British medical school, chat with the medical students and house officers and brush up on his factual knowledge and examinations skills (see Tables 5 and 6). Current examiners usually teach in these medical schools and ask the same questions. This exercise will not only be rewarding, but also enjoyable.

Table 5 Key to success

A. FACTUAL KNOWLEDGE:
- know something about everything
- and everything about something.

B. MEDICAL JARGON:
- English language
- hold a good conversation.

C. EXAMINATION SKILLS:
- demonstrate undergraduate and
- postgraduate training.

D. BRITISH CULTURE:
- appreciate cultural differences
- get to know colloquial English
- understand the structure of the NHS
  and committees.

E. RULES OF THE GAME:
- appreciate British sportsmanship
- don't take failure personally – try again.

Table 6 Sources of information

(Knowledge + jargon + examination skills)

1. Books: A. Undergraduate
                 B. Postgraduate

2. Courses: A. Refresher
                 B. Examination
                 C. Mock exams

3. Training: A. Vocational
                 B. Voluntary

4. Experience   A. General Practice
                 B. Discussion

5. Tips: A. Visit a medical school – learn from final year students.
                 B. Do some postgraduate exams – DCH, DRCOG.

MULTIPLE CHOICE QUESTIONS

Crosswords and quizzes

As a nation, the British like doing jigsaw puzzles, crosswords and quizzes, and playing cards, for pleasure but not necessarily for money. That is why you see so many of these in medical and national journals. This, however, is a blind spot for overseas graduates. In eastern cultures these pastimes are either taboo or frowned upon, and are only done in secret. This is to prevent gambling – if there is a gambler in the family, the whole family are regarded as outcastes for an arranged marriage.

The MCQ paper is a harmless test of factual knowledge covering something about everything. It is certainly not a form of gambling. An overseas graduate should practise doing crosswords and puzzles at least once a week, when they appear in the press.

Trick questions

The English examiners state clearly that there are no trick questions in this examination. Overseas graduates should trust this statement. It is natural for them to expect trickery in examination questions because it is considered very witty by examiners overseas.

Small print

English examiners set questions based on the most common findings of a disease and very rarely set questions on the small print of the textbooks. This is not so in overseas medical schools. The examiners usually ask questions based on the small print in the textbooks, believing that if a candidate can answer such questions, he probably knows the more basic information. An overseas graduate when sitting the MRCGP examination should follow the English custom and stick to the large print.

False sense of security

An MRCGP tutor complained that overseas graduates tried to cheat when marking their own papers in mock examinations. This is false reassurance and there is no point in it. One should sit as many mock examinations as possible and get used to the practice of self-audit – the basis of the MRCGP examination.

MODIFIED ESSAY QUESTION

Unique

The MEQ paper is an invention of the Royal College of General Practitioners. It is a problem-orientated approach to patient care. This is what in fact happens in a GP's surgery. A patient comes in and presents with one problem, the solution of which raises further aspects which need to be investigated and dealt with. There are no definite yes/no answers. Sometimes there are even no answers. But a GP has to deal with each situation as it unfolds. Even British hospital doctors would find it difficult to think along these lines because of their disease-orientated approach, let alone an overseas graduate who perceives the problem as purely a disease entity, the answer to which he thinks can be found in a textbook (see Table 7).

Table 7 Basic English training

---

1. SPEECH AND LANGUAGE:

    Ability to – make oneself understood
                – listen with understanding
                – hold a simple conversation
                – narrate experience
                – discuss and describe environment

2. SOCIAL AND EMOTIONAL:

    Ability to – form appropriate peer relationships
                – communicate with patients
                – accept change and new experience
                – appear relaxed and confident in life situations

3. RESPONSE TO LEARNING SITUATION:

    Ability to – show interest in learning
                – have an inquiring mind
                – persist at a task
                – concentrate on the task in hand
                – manipulate and understand life situations
                – engage in and develop imaginative roleplay

College concept

A patient is seen in the medical model – physical, psychological and social – and in addition emphasis is laid on communication and administrative points. Finally an examiner may ask a few ethical questions. No textbook could cover all these areas completely and an overseas graduate must practise holding a conversation on a patient's problem leading to a discussion and ending up with some recommendations and suggestions. The style of this paper is rather like holding such a discussion.

Religious or scientific approach

Religion is subjectivity and intuition whereas science is objectivity and reason. Therefore there is a significant difference between the two schools of thought (see Table 8). In the MRCGP examination a scientific approach is mandatory. In a mock MEQ paper there was a question: 'Mrs Smith has been delivered of a stillborn child. What exact words would you say to her?' An Arab doctor wrote: 'It is the Will of Allah'. The English tutor gave no marks, but a Muslim examiner would have given full marks. And an Irish or Indian examiner would have given 'grace' marks. It has to be clearly understood that an English examiner thinks scientifically. It is better to be on his wavelength if one wants to pass an English examination.

Table 8 Contradictory concepts: science versus religion

English (Western) – scientific thinking	Overseas (Eastern) – religious approach
Practical	Theoretical
Critical (analytical)	Empirical
Rational	Moral
Unemotional	Emotional

'A' for effort

If an English examiner asks for four causes, he really means four causes. He will not give any marks for extra. In fact, an examiner in an overseas medical school does give marks for extra comments, believing that even if the candidate did not know the answer to **this** question, he has in fact studied the subject, therefore he deserves 'grace' marks. In those countries these 'grace' marks add up and one can still pass the examination without answering the questions precisely. These 'grace' marks are considered to be 'disgrace' marks in Britain, therefore no examiner gives any such marks. He may even be annoyed. Therefore it must be understood that superfluous writing does not pay.

PRACTICE TOPIC QUESTIONS

Essay format

Each question should be answered with a beginning, a middle and an end, because this is what an English examiner expects. In overseas countries, although medical subjects are taught in English, the language itself is not taught as a separate subject. Films and newspapers are in the languages of the country, therefore there is no opportunity to practise using the English language outside the medical schools. This language gap becomes obvious to an English examiner who, of course, gives no 'grace' marks.

Keep it brief

Brevity is the soul of wit. An English graduate is taught from childhood to say a lot in a few words. By the time he reaches medical school, he has learnt to read widely, write briefly and speak succinctly. I wish this was the case in overseas countries! Through no fault of his own, the overseas graduate suffers from this lack of training. He must make up for this deficiency.

Stress of translation

An overseas graduate has the strain of working in two languages, the one, his mother tongue which he speaks with his family at home and has been using with patients of his own ethnic group, and the other, of course, speaking to English patients and colleagues. An English examiner expects him to be as fluent in writing English as an English graduate. Each language has its own restrictions and some phrases just cannot be translated. It is this difficulty which causes him loss of marks, and he should not attribute this to prejudice.

English eyes

I believe it is within the reach of an overseas graduate, who is capable of learning so much scientific knowledge, to improve his essay writing skills by practising at home. He should aim to write in such a way that his written English reads as English to English eyes.

LOG DIARY ORAL

English ears

Ideally an overseas graduate should speak English which sounds English to English ears. If this is not possible, then his or her pronunciation and vocal quality should be such that what is said is clearly understood by the British examiner. I suggest that a candidate should speak slowly, clearly and reasonably loudly. It is not uncommon for an Irish graduate to speak very fast and finish what he wants to say before the examiner has started listening! An Afro-Caribbean or Anglo-Indian, especially a Christian, believes his mother tongue is English but this should not give him a false sense of security. In fact his accent may be very hard to understand to the English examiner. An overseas graduate should always look at the examiner's face and check whether what he is saying is being understood. If there is any doubt, he should ask the examiner politely if he should repeat the answer.

Eye to eye contact

This should be constant during a conversation. In eastern cultures, after an initial glance, it is essential to look away as a gesture of respect. Of course the reverse is the case with the British, where lack of eye to eye contact appears very rude, and symbolises shiftiness or untrustworthiness. If, due to cultural shyness, an overseas graduate is unable to look the English examiner in the eye, perhaps he should look at another part of the examiner's face, such as the nose! However, a German candidate should avoid the piercing eye to eye staring so characteristic of his countrymen.

Over- or understatement

An Englishman has the habit of understatement, whereas an American or Asian is used to boasting. This can become a trap in the log diary oral. An overseas graduate may mention some new expensive equipment which he has bought, to impress the examiner. However, the examiner may question him closely about its use and he could be in trouble if he does not know how to use it. A statement by an overseas graduate that: 'I always take throat swabs before starting an antibiotic' will be regarded very suspiciously by the English examiner, who is ever mindful of the need to cut costs in the NHS.

Absolute honesty

An overseas graduate will religiously collect fifty consecutive cases, whereas an English candidate will omit one or two cases of rare occurrence about which he knows very little. An examiner expects the candidate to discuss each case he or she mentions. There is no hard and fast rule about it but a tactless doctor is a tactless general practitioner, and tact is all-important in this profession.

A patient's wishes

An overseas graduate is trained to think in the patient's interests whereas a British graduate is trained to pay more attention to the patient's wishes in making a decision. For example, if a patient has cancer and he wants to know about it, an English doctor will tell him the truth, accept that the patient will be upset and then give him comfort and counselling. On the other hand, an overseas-trained doctor will try to avoid informing the patient in case he gets upset. In some cultures only the doctor decides. And the patient has to obey his doctor's orders. In the MRCGP examination the English approach must be adopted, not only when treating a British patient but also when dealing with an ethnic minority patient because that is what the English examiner expects.

Difference of opinion

In eastern cultures a difference of opinion is taken too personally. It is not uncommon for an English examiner to say to an overseas graduate: 'I do not agree'. This will be interpreted by the candidate to mean that the examiner is annoyed and therefore he will fail. He will become more and more nervous as a result, and do badly. In English society, freedom of speech is a basic human right. Therefore if someone says 'I do not agree' it does not mean that he is annoyed, only that he has a different point of view. There are some desirable and undesirable attitudes which, in keeping with the British population, are practised by British examiners (see Tables 9 and 10).

Table 9 Orals: desirable attitudes

Openness
Self-awareness
Sensitivity
Confidentiality
Tolerance
Patience
Supportiveness
Enquiring mind
Ability to withstand attack
Self-reliance in patient care
Loyalty to colleagues and patients
Willingness to continue learning
Positive attitude to the College

Table 10 Orals: undesirable attitudes

Rigid (narrow)
Authoritarian
Unselfcritical
Lack of affect
Inconsiderate

Source: Keith Thompson, Examiner, speaking at the MRCGP 6th Annual Study Day for Overseas Graduates, 1983, held at the College.

PROBLEM-SOLVING ORAL

First impressions

An overseas graduate should introduce himself with a smile, be polite, have a sense of humour and be forthcoming. Many such graduates have a built-in fear and suspicion of British examiners. This feeling should be controlled and, given that they possess the correct factual knowledge, examination skills and the right attitude acceptable to British patients, the examiner will be very fair, helpful and willing to pass the candidate. He must give the examiner a chance.

Defensive attitude

It is not uncommon for an overseas graduate to enter the examination room with a defensive attitude rather like a child who has been sent to the headmaster! He may be afraid to open his mouth in case he puts his foot in it! He dreads speaking in front of authority and the examiner has to drag the information out of him. This will not gain him any marks and he will do well to adopt the English graduate's attitude of being forthcoming with the answers and talking in a lively and entertaining manner so that both he and the examiner can enjoy the encounter.

The examiner is never wrong

An overseas graduate told me that he failed the examination because of some transcultural factors, including his belief that an examiner or anyone in a position of authority should not be told to his face that he is wrong. An examiner said to him "I do not visit the elderly because I believe it is a waste of time. I would rather devote this time to preventive clinics. You have shown a lot of night calls visiting the elderly in your Log Diary. Do you think I am a bad GP?" The overseas graduate replied: "No sir, you are not wrong, but perhaps I am". The examiner, interpreted this answer to mean that the candidate was unable to defend himself against attack. This is an undesirable attitude and in borderline cases can result in failure. In eastern cultures a person never disagrees with someone in a position of authority, such as his father, teacher, examiner or income tax officer! This is not the case in Britain and a candidate should feel free to speak his mind as long as he is able to justify his statements.

Irritating habits

There are some habits which are acceptable in one culture but totally unacceptable in another. In eastern cultures, a junior member of a family is not allowed to speak in front of his seniors in the family hierarchy, so he or she speaks out whenever a chance arises, and because time is limited, the speech is very fast, monotonous and argumentative. In English society a person speaks with self-discipline and expresses himself briefly. The other person listens carefully without interrupting the speaker because he will get his turn. The examiner should not get annoyed with an overseas graduate who interrupts him or completes his sentences, because this is a cultural difference (see Table 11). A polite request not to interrupt is all that is needed. However, by realising that he has made a mistake, the candidate may become very worried and the examiner should reassure him, thereby allowing the discussion to continue.

Culturally contentious issues

All the people cannot agree on all the issues all the time. It is natural to have different views on any issue held by followers of different religions and members of different cultures or sub-cultures. An English examiner should not expect that

Table 11 Irritating habits

Nose, ear or tooth-picking
Finger-cracking
Belching
Yawning or coughing without covering the mouth
Foot or leg-shaking
Covering face with hand
Fidgeting
Constant throat-clearing and other small noises
Sneezing without using handkerchief
Sucking sweets, chewing gum or cardomum
Lack of eye-to-eye contact
Speaking halfway through listening
Completing examiner's sentences

---

an overseas graduate will hold the same opinion as he does unless the College has taken up the responsibility of educating such candidates. On the other hand, an overseas graduate, trained in a commonwealth country, should not feel that his view is wrong. It is just different. However, 'when in Rome, do as the Romans do'. A foreign graduate should not be afraid to conform to the examiner's school of thought and at the same time to put forward his own views. As long as both views are expressed, a candidate will not fail. The discussion should be general and never allowed to become personal. Some common topics of a contentious nature are listed in Table 12.

Table 12 Culturally contentious issues

Alcohol
Abortion
Homosexuality
Sexual problems
Unmarried mothers
Mixed marriages
Rectal examination
Naming of the genital organs
Family structure
Place of woman in society
Treatment of elderly parents
Religious convictions or taboos
Personal or shared privacy
National politics
Private practice

LANGUAGE

What English?

"The English have really everything in common with the Americans except of course the language." (Oscar Wilde). Some writers even comment that American

English can be harmful to English ears. Almost everywhere in non-white commonwealth countries the English language is taught by non-English teachers, and the schools do not have language laboratory facilities for creating the proper accents. English knowledge is based on literature rather than the vernacular. Moreover, some British examiners have not had the opportunity to talk to people form other cultures. Under these circumstances an overseas graduate should do his utmost to speak in a way which can be understood by the examiner. He will not fail because of a different accent but he will fail if he is unable to make himself understood. Goodwill on both sides is essential (see Table 13).

Specific words

In some languages words such as 'the' and 'please' do not exist. Some overseas graduates pronounce 'v' as 'w' (ethnic Asians) and 'r' as 'l' (ethnic Chinese). Some Europeans have difficulty pronouncing 'd' and 'th'. If they are sitting an English examination they should try to be aware of this and make a positive effort to be understood. They should not forget to use 'please' when it is due. The improper use of 'the' can change the meaning of a sentence. If the candidate is aware of these differences and points them out to the examiner, the latter will make a special effort to understand him.

Table 13 Recommended reading

---

1. Parkinson, J.E. (1976). *A Manual of English for the Overseas Doctor*, 2nd Edn. Churchill Livingstone
2. Pappworth, M.H. (1975). *Passing Medical Examinations*. Butterworths
3. Hawkins, J. *et al.* (1965). *How Not to Fail the Finals*. J.A. Churchill Ltd.
4. Gambrill, E. and Moulds, A.J. (1984). *Passing the MRCGP*. Pulse
5. Moulds, A.J. *et al.* (1978). *The MRCGP Examination: A Comprehensive Guide to Preparation and Passing*. MTP Press
6. Smith, D.J. (1980). *Overseas Doctors in the National Health Service*. Policy Studies Institute

---

Non-verbal communication

Gestures have different meanings in different cultures. An overseas graduate may be in the habit of waving his index finger while emphasising a point. An English woman examiner will feel particularly insulted because it is considered rude in English culture. It is wiser to avoid counting on the fingers in front of an English examiner because an overseas graduate may inadvertently start showing a reversed 'V' sign. There are many such examples responsible for transcultural misunderstanding.

THINKING

Conflicting views

In my opinion the Royal College of General Practitioners holds the view that all health professionals and patients are British or British-like, and if not, they ought to be. At the moment they do not recognise the differing needs of ethnic minority doctors and patients. On the other hand, overseas graduates feel that they are trained in British-style medical schools, their qualifications are recognised by the General Medical Council, they are in a better position to look after their own ethnic groups and the English law allows them to feel free to practise their religions and cultural attitudes, so why should they be denied entry to the membership of a national body. This makes them feel very bitter. In my opinion this situation, if allowed to persist, will harm both parties and the discipline of general practice. If both sides exercise a little give and take, the future of general practice will benefit.

Right or wrong?

British examiners think in terms of right, wrong and neutral. They perceive various degrees of right and wrong and even if something is wrong, it still has the right to exist. On the other hand, overseas graduates are brought up to believe in the religious terms 'good' and 'bad'. And what is bad must not be allowed to exist. In the MRCGP examination it is not realised by either of the parties that they are speaking two different languages and are not on the same wavelength. In fact they can annoy each other. This situation could be improved by better understanding.

Use your own thoughts

An overseas graduate is in the habit of making broad statements using proverbs and quotations. He will also frequently refer to big textbooks and mention the names of eminent authors. Consequently, the examiner will be left with the impression that he is unable to think for himself. If a candidate praises the College, mentioning for example the Chairman of Council especially, hoping to get more marks, he may in fact end up irritating the examiner who dislikes name-dropping. In fact, an English graduate or examiner has been taught to think in 'role-play' – a situation developing in imagination as if constructing a play – and expects the overseas graduate to join him in this game. This is not something the overseas graduate will find in any book, and it is something he must practise and learn from English colleagues, as indeed, his English colleagues will learn from him.

CONCLUSION

The contents of this chapter are directed at both British and overseas graduates, and their examiners. My aim is not to patronise or denigrate anyone but to identify and quantify the cultural differences involved and to suggest ways of bridging these gaps. Transcultural understanding, I believe, is essential and is a step forward in British general practice in making it more appropriate to the needs of the whole of the British nation.

Sixth Annual Study Day for Overseas Graduates

For the last six years the North and West London faculty has organized an annual study day for overseas graduates who are preparing to sit the MRCGP examination. Responsibility for the course has always rested with the Education Committee of the Faculty and for the last two years the course organizer has been Dr Bashir Qureshi.

The MRCGP pass rate for overseas graduates is lower than that for those who have qualified in the UK. Hence the need to study the special problems of overseas graduates was identified by the Committee. The Study Day aims to familiarize potential candidates with the format and style of the MRCGP examinations, and also provides a forum for sharing experiences and forming study groups. Moreover, it provides opportunities to look at problems in communication between patient and doctor as well as those between examiner and candidate, in order to encourage those with difficulties to work on them and improve their skills.

The first Study Day was held in 1977 and each year it has been an astounding success. This year there were 189 applicants but only 100 could be accepted. Study Day tutors included College examiners, faculty members and an English teacher. The format of the day varied from short talks by the examiners on various parts of the examination to work in small groups.

Learning has been two-way, for by having first-hand experience of the cultural difficulties of some of their candidates, the examiners themselves may become more understanding of them.

The replies of participants to evaluation questionnaires for the day have indicated that once again this event has been highly appreciated. Perhaps there is a need for other faculties to hold Study Days such as those for overseas graduates. The Education Committee of the North and West London Faculty plans another such day for 11 February 1984.

First published in *J. Roy. Coll. Gen. Practit.*, **33**(251), June 1983, pp.381–382 (Royal College of General Practitioners)

Seventh annual study day for overseas graduates

One-fifth of all practising general practitioners in the United Kingdom are overseas graduates, looking after about ten million British patients. Of these, only a handful have been able to pass the MRCGP examination (about 5% in 1981). It is essential for good patient care that the standard for this examination remains high. If overseas-trained general practitioners can be brought up to this standard by further education, this would be a great service to British patients, and it is encouraging that the pass rate for overseas graduates had risen to about 25% in 1983.

The North and West London Faculty was the first faculty to be aware of this situation. Its education committee runs courses for member and non-member general practitioners and also for specific groups which it considers need special attention. In keeping with this policy, the Seventh Annual Study Day for Overseas Graduates was held at 14 Princes Gate on Saturday, 11th February 1984. This was heavily oversubscribed with more than 200 applicants. The original intention was to accept a maximum of 100 candidates but the demand was such that the figure had to be raised to 110, though in the event 90 actually attended. Of the 13 tutors, nine were examiners, three were faculty members and one an English language teacher. The examiners were Drs Andrew Bailey, John Cohen, John Lee (Chairman of the Membership Division), Michael Lee-Jones, Cameron Lockie, Bill Marson, Peter Mukherji, Lotte Newman and John Toby. The faculty members included Drs George Melotte, Jayant Thakkar and myself, and the English teacher was John Clegg. This very strong team was extremely well equipped to deal with all aspects of the cultural and educational problems facing overseas graduates preparing for the MRCGP examination.

The syllabus consisted of work in small groups covering various parts of the examination, but dealing particularly with the problems encountered by overseas graduates, and talks by examiners and teachers covering not only the examination and general practice but also an introduction to the College and job prospects in general practice. The quality of care of these general practitioners was considered as important as the quality of care in general practice.

The rapport between the examiners and the candidates was so good that the organiser found it difficult to break up these small groups in order to start the final plenary session. At this session, and in the 67 questionnaires returned, the candidates asked for repeat, extended and frequent study days of this type. Although the problem was originally identified by the home faculty, it is recognised that this is a national issue and there is a need for other faculties to hold such courses in their postgraduate centres.

An analysis of attendance showed that the majority of the candidates were already general practitioner principals; some were trainees, and there was a handful of locums. There was also one English trainer attending to help him teach overseas trainees. There were no hospital doctors.

This study day was unique in three respects. First, the candidates were able to discuss their educational and cultural difficulties directly with the College examiners, and benefit from their advice, a contact which has already raised the

First published in *1984 RCGP Members' Reference Book*, p.119 (Royal College of General Practitioners)

pass percentage of these candidates in the past two years. Secondly, the examiners were able to reassure the candidates that there was no colour prejudice in this examination, as might have been believed. The College aims at membership by inclusion and not by exclusion and its scientific thinking was explained by the organiser who also gave advice on the cultural differences which were acting as a barrier for borderline candidates. Finally, the English participants came to understand the overseas graduates' viewpoints and appreciated their determination to become better general practitioners. Specific problems were identified and ways of dealing with them were established, and the day ended on a note of optimism for the future.

North and West London Faculty eighth annual study day for overseas graduates

Cultural differences in science are well respected. British general practitioners come from many different cultures, as do their patients. Learning behaviour, test performance and the quality of medical practice inevitably vary with a person's beliefs and training. The College promotes postgraduate education for all general practitioners, conducts the membership examination and strives to ensure high standards of practice. In medical thinking there is no place for discrimination – negative or positive – but a fair distinction between each patient's ethnic, religious and cultural needs is essential. Different needs require different answers. A provider of health care needs the appropriate education to enable him to serve all consumers. To identify such needs, the North and West London Faculty holds an annual study day for overseas graduates.

Limited Section 63 funds placed the study day in doubt. However, the feedback from past years was such that we could not cancel it, but had to accept a reduction in numbers.

Learning and teaching go hand in hand. At the study day the teachers and the candidates learn from each other. College examiners become teachers; this is a demonstration that the College believes in membership by inclusion and not by exclusion. The College is not only concerned with those who pass the examination, but also assist those who do not reach the required standard but are willing to try and achieve it by continued education.

At the time of writing we are in the final stages of planning this year's annual study day. The teaching staff consist of eight College examiners and three faculty course organizers. The examiners are Drs John Lee, (Chairman, Membership Division), Andrew Bailey, Peter Burrows, Cameron Lockie, Peter Mukherji, Lotte Newman, George Taylor and John Toby. The faculty members are Drs George Melotte (Faculty Chairman), Jayant Thakkar and myself.

First published in *J. Roy. Coll. Gen. Practit.*, **35**(275), June 1985, p.306 (Royal College of General Practitioners)

The programme begins with an introduction to the College and then covers various parts of the examination, dealing particularly with the problems encountered by overseas graduates – educational as well as cultural. Various talks by examiners and teachers cover most aspects of general practice, including job prospects.

The objectives of this study day are:

- To familiarize potential candidates with the format and style of the MRCGP examination.
- To identify some of the special problems of overseas graduates who take the examination, in order to help them prepare for it appropriately.
- To look at problems in communication between patient and doctor as well as between examiner and candidate, in order to encourage those with difficulties to improve their skills.
- To provide a forum for sharing experiences and an opportunity to form study groups.

CHAPTER 23

MUSLIM PATIENTS AND THE BRITISH GP

INTRODUCTION

Science has to do with objectivity and reason whereas religion has to do with subjectivity and intuition. At first sight they seem incompatible: the scientific approach is practical, analytical, critical and unemotional, whereas the religious approach is theoretical, empirical, moral and emotional. The British general practitioner is primarily a scientist yet may well be deeply religious, and his patient too may be deeply religious and yet be a scientist. No one can be pigeon-holed precisely and not all situations can be judged by the same yardstick. Few patients present as textbook cases; every clinical picture tells a different story.

Avoiding the politics of integration and segregation, I have studied transcultural medicine in the UK for twenty years and tried to assess the problems encountered in consultations between doctors and patients of different ethnic groups, cultures and religions. A problem can be medical (physical, psychological, social) cultural or religious, or a combination of any of these. This chapter discusses the religious problems which can affect the British general practitioner in relation to his Muslim patients.

There are three reasons why a general practitioner should learn about the interface between medicine and the Muslim religion:

1. The need to allay the fear of the unknown.
2. The need to provide health care for the whole community rather than just a section of it.
3. The need to match individual patient's demands with the demands of society.

WHAT IS ISLAM?

Islam is based on five principles:

1. The belief in one God or Allah and in Mohammed His Messenger, to whom He revealed the Holy Qur'an (Koran), the Holy Book of Muslims.

First published in *The Medical Annual 1984*, pp.259–271 (John Wright/Institute of Physics)

2. Namaz – prayer five times daily, facing in the direction of the Holy Mosque at Mecca.
3. Ramadan – fasting for one lunar month (Islamic calender) every year.
4. Compulsory Zakat (poor dues) for the benefit of the needy – 2.5 per cent of a Muslim's total bank balance and property value, which is paid once a year.
5. Haj – a pilgrimage to Mecca at least once in a lifetime, if the journey can be undertaken.

Medicine in society

The word 'Allah' is the Arabic for God and Muslims do not like it to be translated into other languages, to avoid misinterpretation. General practitioners should remember this. Mohammed is the name of the prophet who preached equality to mankind and discouraged hero worship so strongly that no Muslim will allow an image, picture or statue to be made of him. Some Muslims learn the Holy Qur'an by heart to recite in the Holy Month of Ramadan at the time of evening prayer – such a person is called a Hafiz. The Islamic Holy Day is Friday, therefore a general practitioner can expect more consultations on that day.

The mosque is a place of worship which is built and run by the local Muslim community. It is unique in that not only is it a place to say prayers but it also provides a free evening meal for anyone attending the evening prayer session and free overnight accomodation for Muslim travellers (although some mosques may not have these facilities). Therefore a general practitioner who comes across a homeless or hungry Muslim can suggest that he goes to the local mosque. Moreover, a non-Muslim in the same circumstances can also be helped, provided the doctor contacts the mosque, because a non-Muslim would not then be expected to pray in the Muslim fashion. No fee is charged because all expenses are paid by the local Muslim community. Thus a stable network of support is available for the general practitioner with Muslim patients and he may benefit from paying a visit to the local mosque and meeting the local Muslim community.

The Imam is a religious leader and counsellor of the Muslim community. He is chosen for his knowledge and skill in religious and related affairs, and plays the part of a 'caretaker'. He lives near the mosque and is responsible for the religious, social, educational, economic and health welfare of Muslims. He will therefore be happy to help if contacted and normally has a positive attitude towards general practitioners. Primary care has become multidisciplinary and general practitioners have been using the services of carers such as marriage guidance counsellors for some time. Thus, where appropriate, there is no reason not to use the Imam as another resource and consult him as frequently as any other religious leader. Good communication, consultation and conference are essential for a general practitioner's role in society.

The Islamic calender is based on lunar months. A lunar month can be 29 or 30 days long, but never 28 or 31 days. The Islamic year is 355 days long (not 365): seven 30-day months and five 29-day months. For example, Ramadan will start ten days earlier in each Christian year – in 1986 Ramadan started on 14 May; in 1987 it started on 4 May, in 1988 on 24 April and in 1989 on 14 April. Ramadan occurs in the same Christian month only once every 36 Christian years. In his lifetime a Muslim is likely to see only one winter and one summer Ramadan. This information is important to the general practitioner, not only in relation to the time when Ramadan fasting takes place, but when a Muslim patient describes his age.

If a good doctor – patient relationship is to be achieved, appropriate greetings are essential. A male Muslim likes to shake hands and say 'Assalamu-alaikum' which means 'Peace be upon you'. A Muslim woman will say the same words but will not wish to shake hands with the doctor. It will therefore save embarrassment if the doctor can remember this. Women doctors should also be sensitive to the shock that may be suffered by a Muslim man on being confronted by a female doctor.

MUSLIMS IN THE UK

There are about two million Muslims in Britain and 515 mosques with attached schools. These Muslims are originally from Pakistan, Bangladesh, the Arab countries, Iran, Turkey, Indonesia and Malaysia. All Muslims have one thing in common with the British: they are devoted to business and willing to travel for this purpose. A general practitioner can feel free to have a general chat on business affairs: nevertheless it cannot be over-emphasized that all Muslims do not come from the same culture and cultural differences can affect the course of an illness. The Islamic Centre, near Baker Street, London, has a big library where non-Muslims can get more information. The librarian is usually a theological scholar and any doctor can ring him if he has a query. An Imam is also attached to the premises.

Muslims modify their religious customs to British needs; for example in Muslim countries, the call to prayer in every mosque is relayed over a loud speaker, called an Azaan (call), but in Britain this is not observed in the same way in order to adapt to British society. If a general practitioner or any non-Muslim has any reason to complain, he should not hesitate to contact the local Imam from whom he can expect a favourable response.

RELIGIOUS DUTIES

The duties which can affect the general practitioner include Ramadan fasting, Namaz (prayers) and Haj (pilgrimage to Mecca) – see Table 1.

Ramadan

The month of Ramadan is the ninth month of the Muslim calender. Every year, Muslims observe fasting during this month every day from dawn to dusk. They believe that fasting has many advantages, including self-discipline, variation from the daily routine, time for prayer to strengthen willpower, dieting and keeping fit. Many beauticians of all religions attribute the secret of a healthy skin and physical fitness to fasting one day a week.

Each fast day starts at sunrise and ends at sunset, the length of the day depending on the country and the time of year. In 1983, the fasting day started at about 3 a.m. and ended at about 9.30 p.m.

The majority of devout Muslims happily accept this long period of fasting. They are expected to work as usual – fasting is not regarded as an excuse to take time off from work or school. During fasting, they are not allowed to eat, drink (not even water), smoke, use an inhaler or have injections. They are not allowed to use toothpaste, nor to insert ear- or nose-drops. A married couple is expected to abstain from any sexual contact during the fasting day. A meal is taken before sunrise (Sehri) and the fast is broken at sunset, usually with dates (a religious custom) or a proper meal, and then prayers are said. The day after the end of Ramadan is celebrated as a festival and is known as Eid Day. This is the equivalent of Christmas Day in importance.

Table 1 Health value of the rituals

Ritual	Physical	Psychological	Social	Relevance for general practitioner
Ramadan fasting	Increased stamina Slimming	Self-discipline Willpower	Family togetherness Eid Festival – family reconciliations	Exemption certificates Drug compliance
Prayers (5 times a day)	Exercise Washing (self)	Self-audit Psychotherapy	Community spirit Short breaks from stress of work	Less mental illness Reassurances to employers about ritual
Pilgrimage to Mecca (once in a lifetime)	Travel Circulation of money Better nutrition	Stimulation Sense of achievement	International exchange of views and business contracts	Immunizations Tropical health problems

A general practitioner attached to a factory where Muslims are employed needs to know that these employees are expected to work as usual and do not need refreshment breaks, though they certainly need time for prayers. A factory worker may opt to do night shifts, if this is acceptable.

Fasting will inevitably cause hypoglycaemia, thus reducing some efficency at work, but prayer should strengthen willpower and self-discipline, and result in increased productivity in other areas.

An occupational health nurse may be approached by Muslim staff for minor ailments such as fatigue or feeling hot or weak. In fact such an employee is seeking sympathy and reassurance. All that is necessary is supportive counselling and encouragement to carry on working – advice that he or she will gladly follow.

Children are expected to observe fasting from the age of 12. They fast initially for a few days, and then for the whole month as they become older. A doctor attached to a school health service or a welfare assistant in a school may be approached by children who cannot tolerate fasting for the whole day. In such cases the fast can be broken and school work allowed to continue, but the pupil is asked to tell his parents about this. Such incidents should not be frowned upon and the child's faith should be respected.

Usually a general practitioner likes to have a brief social chat before examining the patient and a much better rapport can be established by chatting about Ramadan when appropriate, rather than about the usual topics such as sport, holidays or business.

Exemption. General practitioners may be asked to give medical certificates for exemption from fasting. Muslims are exempt from fasting during illness or long-distance travel. Women are exempt during menstruation and are not allowed to pray at this time. However, they have to make up the fasting days after their menstruation.

Second and third generation Muslims may lapse in their observance of Ramadan and may have feelings of guilt, particularly if first generation Muslims show disapproval of their lack of self-discipline. They may also have some other hidden vice such as drinking or smoking. Such a 'lapsed' person may present with vague, exaggerated or invented complaints in the hope that his doctor will prescribe medication and give a sick note, which he can show to his family. Care should be taken to see that genuine patients are not mistaken for such patients.

A patient may be reluctant to ask for exemption but hope to get it. In a complicated situation the doctor should give medical advice and then ask the patient to see his Imam for religious clarification. He may also like to contact the Imam himself. An asthmatic who needs an inhaler or an unstable diabetic would be ill enough to qualify for exemption, and a general practitioner should not hesitate to exempt ill patients from fasting, and make the suggestion himself where appropriate.

Medical conditions

Indigestion. Some Muslims may overeat at Sehri (the meal before sunrise) in anticipation of the next day's fasting. They may also go straight to bed after eating instead of staying up to pray as they should. Some may even have more spices in their food than usual. All these factors can lead to indigestion, and during Ramadan, general practitioners will do well to anticipate this.

Insomnia. Adults or children may complain of sleep disturbances, especially in the early days of Ramadan fasting. Simple reassurance may be sufficient.

Nutritional disorders. Some Muslims live in rented accomodation, sharing kitchen facilities with English tenants, who may find Sehri cooking inconvenient; in order not to disturb their neighbours, the Muslims may resort to tinned or 'junk' food, or even go without their one meal. Such families may present problems of undernutrition and malnutrition. In severe cases this can lead to nutritional anaemias.

Diabetes. As with other medical diets, fasting may conflict with the regimes of patients on diabetic or reducing diets, and in acute cases a medical certificate may exempt them from fasting. A local Imam may be contacted and will support the doctor's advice.

Prescribing during Ramadan. To achieve full compliance, the doctor should ask the patient to be frank in discussing any fears he may have on medicine conflicting with his religious beliefs during this time of increased religious awareness. Medicines containing alcohol and pork-derived insulin should not be prescribed, especially during Ramadan.

The times for oral medication are sunset, before retiring, and at Sehri. Wherever possible, such drugs, especially antibiotics, should be prescribed in once or twice daily dosage, rather than three or four times a day, which may lead to partial or non-compliance.

Prayers

There are five prayer sessions of 20 to 30 minutes' duration: at sunrise, after lunch, late afternoon (tea-time), sunset and before retiring. During office hours (9 a.m. to 5 p.m.) a worker may need a prayer-break after lunch and at tea-time, usually no more than half an hour. The prayers at sunrise, sunset and late evening are, of course, not in working hours. Each prayer session consists of a physical exercise, recitation of the Holy Qur'an, and relaxation of the mind.

At the time of prayer, a Muslim gets a chance for self-audit, peer audit and consultation with an Imam or his colleagues. For someone under duress, the prayer session may serve as autotherapy if he is praying alone, individual psychotherapy if he is consulting an Imam and group therapy if he is praying with fellow workers or neighbours.

Two medical conditions are worth considering by a general practitioner. First, some people who pray for long periods of time develop callosities on their forehead and ankles, and come to the doctor for treatment. However, some will come just for self-reassurance and will not ask for treatment. Secondly, since the prayers are a form of relaxation therapy, very occasionally one can expect 'meditation catatonia'.

Haj – pilgrimage to Mecca

It is the life-long ambition of every Muslim to make a pilgrimage to Mecca and the Holy Shrine of the Prophet Mahommed in Medina in Saudi Arabia. A Muslim may consult his doctor to have the appropriate inoculations for his family and himself, and for recommendations regarding prophylactic medication before travelling. He may express his anxieties about long-distance travel and want a chat with his family doctor.

Sometimes he makes his pilgrimage in the summer, when the weather is extremely hot in Saudi Arabia. Rarely, he may contract a tropical disease when abroad, but boils due to heat are more common. These boils, even when healed, leave scars which should not be mistaken for something more sinister. It is customary to bring some tinned food or holy water from the holy spring (called Zamzam). During travel, refrigeration facilities may not be of a very high standard and there is the possibility of *Salmonella typhimurium* food poisoning, and very rarely, typhoid fever or meningococcal menigitis. A general practitioner should be actively on the look-out for this. A Muslim family would be delighted to be offered a medical check by their doctor on their return to exclude any infection.

RELIGIOUS BELIEFS

Allah-the-healer

A Muslim believes that Allah is Shafi (the Healer) and that it is He who provides the cure for an illness. A Muslim believes that Allah gives the general practitioner the power to think of the correct diagnosis and treatment. He believes in fate and the Will of Allah to an extent that he will accept any consequence of the disease or treatment that may follow. He believes that Satan can misguide a person, but not that he causes illness. Therefore, any belief such as a person being possessed is a cultural phenomenon and not a religious belief. A doctor can expect better results if he tells a Muslim 'Allah will cure you'. This phrase will have a magic effect on such a patient, who will be very appreciative. The peace of mind which can result from this doctor – patient rapport can only have a beneficial effect on his illness.

Sanctity of life

Another firm belief of Muslims is a conviction of the sanctity of life: killing is always wrong, no matter what the circumstances. Suicide, abortion and euthanasia are forbidden in Islam. However, a hunger strike as a means of protest or dying in the cause of Islam are considered as martyrdom. Holy War – Jehad – is defined and declared by a Chief Imam of a country, and only in those circumstances is dying considered sacred. A general practitioner can contact an Imam in two situations: first if a patient refuses to take a medicine which the doctor believes is life-saving, and secondly, if he has to attend a patient on a hunger strike which has not been declared as Jehad.

RELIGIOUS CUSTOMS

Purdah

A Muslim woman must wear a veil when coming into contact with a man who is not a member of her extended family, and this includes the doctor. This custom is observed by all Muslim women, though less strictly in Britain. The philosophy is 'The less you know of others, the more you will stick to one'. This is to guard marriage and family life. It may conflict with the western philosophy of 'Try before you buy', which ensures freedom of choice, a basic human right very dear to the British.

There are two things which will concern the general practitioner in relation to purdah. First, a woman patient will be very nervous or even frightened of being examined by a male doctor. She may never have been touched by a man, apart from her husband, and a physical examination may be seen as a great threat. It is almost impossible to establish a good rapport in such circumstances, especially for a gynaecological examination. It is folly to try to treat a Muslim woman just like an English woman because her needs are so different. The problem can usually be overcome by counselling or compromise, unless the examination is essential to save life, in which case the husband or Imam can be asked to help.

British governments have maintained that allocating women doctors for women patients is an act of sex discrimination. This is very much a western point of view which is not understood in the east, so the British general practitioner should try to be as flexible as possible. If his practice has a woman doctor this will greatly reassure his Muslim women patients, who should be enabled to see her whenever possible.

Secondly, women in purdah may not escort children to and from school while their husbands are at work and their children are then brought home by friends and neighbours. Unfortunately they sometimes show off on the way home to the extent of risking a road accident. Road accidents are recognized as a common cause of death in school children in the UK, and recent evidence suggests that it is more common in Muslim children. A general practitioner interested in social psychology has much to offer in such circumstances.

Circumcision

Female circumcision is not indicated by Islam. It is a cultural issue of ethnic North Africans. However, male circumcision is a compulsory requirement for a Muslim and is usually carried out in the first two years of life. In Muslim countries, the operation is done by barbers, even nowadays. Muslim parents in the United Kingdom find it difficult to decide where to get circumcision done privately. Now that contraceptive devices are prescribed under the NHS, it is time to rethink the possible provision of circumcision under the NHS. After all, it is in everyone's interests to avoid back-street operations.

The scientific reason for circumcision is said to be prevention of phimosis and paraphimosis which may occur in hot weather. Even England can have hot summers, and general practitioners may well be asked to recommend a good and sympathetic surgeon. Florid cases of phimosis or paraphimosis are already treated by circumcision under the NHS.

Halal meat

This is meat from the ritual killing of a live animal and is similar to kosher meat killing for Jews.

Muslim dress

Women wear traditional kurta (a long skirt) and salwar (pyjama trousers). This dress conforms with the philosophy of purdah, since it covers a woman from head to toe. Interestingly it does not interfere with physical education in schools.

It takes longer for a Muslim woman to undress because of cultural shyness and the special dress, and a practice nurse is well advised to be very patient.

Miswak – scented wood

Miswak is a scented wood used by devout Muslims for dental cleansing. Some Muslims may not be used to using toothpaste and toothbrushes. Nevertheless their dental hygiene is likely to be satisfactory because miswak is a good dental brush with a herbal remedy in it to clean teeth adequately. A dental surgeon who does not frown upon this religious custom will not lose these patients.

Fallacy

The idea that a Muslim is allowed four wives is an old wives' tale. It is clear from the heads of state of Muslim countries that they are monogamous. The late Shah of Iran had to divorce Queen Soraya in order to marry Farah Deba. In Islamic history there is but one precedent. After the conquest of Syria and Egypt by Muslims, there were fewer men left to more women (war widows on both sides). A meeting of war veterans decided that each soldier should receive the spoils of war and look after one or two war widows, on the understanding that he treated them as equals of his own wife.

Thus no general practitioner need fear that he has a polygamous patient on his books!

RELIGIOUS TABOOS

Every religion has taboos and Islam is no exception. Islamic taboos include alcohol, pork, statues, images, pictures, photographs, jazz, dogs, crosses, sex education, postmorten examinations and cremation.

Alcohol

Because alcohol affects the power of judgement, the Muslim religion strongly forbids it: an alcoholic may risk an accident, divorce, and the sack. Moreover, 'Alcohol provokes the desire but takes away the performance'. A general practitioner must avoid using medicines which contain alcohol, such as tonics and surgical spirit, even though they are socially accepted in the west. A Muslim patient who sees these things on prescriptions or on the labels of bottles may not complain to his doctor but may feel so disgusted that he may never trust that doctor again. He may find this a reason for turning to alternative medicine.

Pork

Cleanliness is next to godliness. This is a central philosophy of all religions and Islam also abides by it. Symbolism is an important element in religion. Islam chose the pig to be a symbol of uncleanliness because it lives in a sty. A traditional belief that we are what we eat dominates the suspicion of Muslim patients and they detest the thought of eating pork and all its derivatives such as bacon, ham and lard. They are so sensitive on this point that pork insulin should never, ever, be prescribed for a Muslim patient. A patient who is allergic to beef and cannot have pork should be given Humulin insulin. There is a problem here – Humulin insulin has the connotation of being derived from human flesh, and the general practitioner should be sensitive to his patient's fears, even if they are not expressed verbally, and explain that this is synthetic preparation and not made from human flesh. Human insulin derived from pork should also be avoided.

Images, statues, pictures, photographs

Images of any kind are forbidden in Islam because it is thought that they imitate God's creations. Only Allah should create living things and any attempt to make copies is a challenge to his authority. Muslim women sometimes refuse to have a photograph taken, even for a passport. A doctor would be well advised not to take a Muslim friend to visit Madame Tussaud's or the Louvre, and should not expect to be sent picture postcards from Muslim friends on holiday.

Jazz

Music is the food of love and love before marriage is frowned upon in Islam. Therefore, only religious music is allowed. A devout Muslim may politely decline an offer of a cassette from a pharmaceutical company sending him a piece of western music in good faith.

Dogs

Dogs are considered unclean by Muslims, who will not even touch one. The British are a nation of dog lovers but it is wise to avoid the subject when in conversation with a Muslim.

Crosses

The red cross is a historical symbol of Christian armies who fought in Crusades. Muslims are taught history alongside religion and while they may tolerate the red cross symbol on ambulances, as it is so universal, their feelings will be hurt if, in the event of a bereavement, someone sends them a card bearing a Christian cross.

Sex education

Premarital sex and adultery are considered great threats to marriage and family life, institutions held dear by Muslims. To guard them all marriages are arranged.

It is considered offensive by devout Muslim parents to give sex education to unmarried girls.

Postmortem examination

In keeping with respect for the dead, Islam does not allow postmortem examinations. Therefore these should not be undertaken lightly. In medico-legal cases, the police surgeon should have a quiet word with the next of kin or preferably the Imam, who will pray for the deceased and allow this examination only if it is legally binding.

Cremation

Under no circumstances will Muslims allow cremation and they will insist that their dead are buried. This is because they believe in life after death and that the preservation of the body gives consolation to the soul. Muslims value visits to the graves and shrines of their dead for prayers. They venerate these graves, generation after generation.

ALTERNATIVE MEDICINE

Muslim patients use five therapies. These are scientific medicine, religious therapy, faith healing, Hakims' remedies and food therapy. Unfortunately, they often use more than one therapy at the same time.

Religion as therapy

Religion is used as therapy by following a regime of meditation. This can have a hypotensive effect. Therefore a patient on antihypertensive treatment should be asked how much meditation he is doing, and while there is no laboratory test to monitor this, the general practitioner should be in a position to advise about adjusting treatment. To avoid hypotensive episodes, he may have to reduce the dosage of antihypertensive medication.

Faith healing

Faith healing is not advised in Islam but is widely practised by Muslims, perhaps as traditional medicine, and involves the use of charms and amulets. These contain writings of words from the Holy Qur'an with the blessings of a faith healer. This form of therapy is used in varying degrees ranging from mending a broken love affair to treating a chronic illness. A general practitioner may not believe in it, but if he shows any disrespect of a patient's faith, it will damage the relationship, perhaps irreparably. He might even wish his patient good luck; after all, the patient believes in fate!

Hakims' remedies

A Hakim is a Muslim practitioner who uses herbal medicine and perhaiz – the avoidance of certain foods liable to cause allergies (e.g shellfish) or colonic irritation (e.g. red chillies). He may even prescribe kushtas, which are compounds of mercury, or other metals in syrup, wrapped in thin silver fool. These are considered to be aphrodisiacs. The problem is one of metal intoxication; for example, mercury may cause mental instability. To an unwary doctor these symtoms may cause a diagnostic dilemma.

Food therapy

There are many foods which are used in the treatment of common conditions, dates and honey being used by many Muslim patients. Dates relieve constipation and honey is believed to be a panacea.

Alternative medicine may potentiate, counteract or conflict with orthodox treatment, but before he condemns it the general practitioner should remember that although scientific medicine began with the Greeks, there were men who practised the art of healing long before the Greek physicians. In spite of his scientific beliefs, a general practitioner should try to understand his patient's beliefs in alternative medicine and allow him to use them unless they conflict with his own treatment. In such circumstances, dogmatic advice is likely to fall on deaf ears. Understanding, persuasion and regular follow-up will provide the key to success.

CONCLUSION

It is not essential for a British general practitioner to know everything about Islam, but the suggestions made in this section may serve as a useful guide when dealing with Muslim patients in the surgery. If he learns to appreciate the role of an Imam as a counsellor, the role of a mosque as a place of shelter for the homeless, the need of Muslim women for a female doctor, and above all, the need to respect the patient's faith, which may include a belief in alternative medicine, then he will go a long way towards establishing the rapport which is so fundamental to the doctor-patient relationship in general practice.

FURTHER READING

Barber, R. (1983). Society wields the knife and gives a badge for life (Focus on circumcision). *Current Practice*, 4 February, 22-3

Barber, S.G. and Wright, A.D. (1979). Muslims, Ramadan, and diabetes mellitus. Letter. *British Medical Journal*, **2**, 675

Ebbing, R.N. (1979). Muslims, Ramadan, and diabetes mellitus. Letter. *British Medical Journal*, **2**. 333-4

Ferreyra, C. (1979). The immigrant's many problems. *General Practitioner*, 9th March, 19

Henley, A. (1983). Muslim men and women do not share names. *Medeconomics*, 36-41

Kinlen, L.J. (1982). Meat and fat consumption and cancer mortality: a study of strict religious orders in Britain. *Lancet*, **1**, 946-9

Lawrence, C. (1983). Medicine in the Islamic world. *Update*, **27**, 259-66

McKeown, T. and Lowe, C.R. (1974). *Causes of International Differences. An Introduction to Social Medicine*. London, Blackwell Scientific Publications, PP.75-76

Philip, G. (1979). Veiled Saudi women are problem patients in surgery. *Pulse*, 11th August

Ramadan Timetable (1983). Central Jamia Masjid, 12 Pluckington Place, Southall, Middlesex

Ruck, N. (1979). Understanding Asian patients. *General Practitioner*, 9th March, 19

Sarguroh, A.K. (1982). Islam versus democracy. *Daily Jang*, London, 6th November, 5

Shaker, J.J. and Rais, C. (1983). *Mash-hoor Alam Jantari 1983* (Urdu language). Gurg & Co. Booksellers, 484 Kara Bowli, Delhi, India

Singer, C. and Underwood, E.A. (1962). *The Dawn of Medicine: Medicine in Prehistoric Times. A Short History of Medicine*. Oxford, Clarendon Press, pp. 1-15

Udezue, E. (1983). Conspiracy helps take the Pill into purdah. *Doctor*, 19th May, 61

Walton, P. (1982). Muslims say 'No' to sex classes. *Doctor*, 11th March, 68

Wolfe, K. (1983). British religious broadcasting in perspective. *Religious Broadcasting Now*, London, IBA Publications, pp.ix-xi

---

Beware when diagnosing 'battered' Muslim children

Inner-city GPs may be finding themselves called to case conferences to examine 'battered' Muslim children, but they must be wary of this diagnosis.

An average inner-city practice may have 200 Muslim patients. About 50 of these will be Shia Muslims, who have just finished a period of religious devotion that involves considerable self-abuse. Males will beat their chests with slaps and punches resulting in bruising and some devout Shia Muslims may beat their chests and backs with chains, knives and needles in a ritual in front of their peers. Children will begin participating in these ceremonies when they are about 10 and they are often very enthusiastic about their devotions.

A teacher, having noticed bruising in a child, had notified a social worker and that both parties had been loath to believe that the wounds could be self-inflicted. But genuine cases of non-accidental injury should not be overlooked.

A child who is half asleep during lessons will not necessarily be suffering from a TATT syndrome. It is more likely that he attended Majlis (mass) the previous evening and it is a short-term problem which should be tactfully handled.

Religious ritual leaves its mark

Shia Muslims, who stem mainly from Iran, Iraq and Lebanon, may have just finished observing the remembrance ceremonies and rituals to mark the anniversary of the brutal killing of Hazrad Imam Hussein, the grandson of the Prophet Mahommed, in 631 AD.

The ceremonies were conducted over the whole month of Moharram, the first month of the Islamic calendar.

First published in *Pulse*, **44**, No.42, Oct.27 1984, p.43 (Morgan Grampian Professional Press)

In the period of mourning, a Shia Muslim wears black funeral dress. He will go to an Imam Bara (mosque) with his family and attend a religious mass called Majlis, especially in the first 10 days of Moharram.

Some Shia males not only feel grieved but also angry. To release this anger and conduct the bereavement properly, they may beat their chests with slaps and punches, which could result in bruising.

If during an examination a GP notices bruises and scars, he should understand that these are self-inflicted injuries as a result of a holy ritual rather than a psychiatric problem. He should not hesitate to talk about it to the patient.

HAVE A MIND FOR MUSLIM MATTERS

The British GP and Muslim patient is an instance where a good doctor – patient relationship requires particular effort and mutual understanding. A few minor lapses or 'innocent omissions' can so easily damage a tentative doctor – patient rapport. In the event of an 'I'm-sorry-if-I-upset-you, I-didn't-mean-to', things may never be the same again.

The British GP is used to seeing one English patient at a time; even if an English mother accompanies her child, the doctor will ask the child a direct question. This is not the case with Muslim patients.

In keeping with their extended family system, the head of the family will take time off work to bring a member of his family who needs to see the doctor. And to avoid frequent absences from work, he will bring the whole family, just in case other members need attention. He will speak for the family and, in his absence, the family hierarchy is maintained – a mother speaks for her children, an older sibling may give the history on behalf of a younger one.

This should not irritate an understanding GP. If he wishes to ask a member of the family to give his or her own history, he should tell the head of the family, who will cooperate happily. Although this may increase the volume of work at a particular GP consultation, it will in fact reduce further separate consultations and home visits. Teaching practices believing in patient participation however, should modify their consultations accordingly.

In keeping with the arranged marriage concept and purdah in the Muslim faith, men are segregated from women, even at the time of saying prayers. No disrespect is intended if a male patient asks to be examined by a male doctor, and similarly, a Muslim woman will insist on seeing a female doctor. It is certainly not an act of sex discrimination but, as a byproduct, it increases the chances of employment for women doctors.

Doctors should, too, respect certain customs and religious practices. A GP trainee expects that a child's prepuce should not be retracted before the age of two years, but he should not show surprise when he sees a Muslim infant who

First published in *GP*, June 29 1984, p.21 (Medical Publications Ltd)

has been circumcised, as this is an extremely important religious ritual. And it is customary for Muslim men and women to shave their pubic hair. This may surprise some English doctors who are not used to this custom, but it should not be commented on.

A Muslim patient will refuse to see a psychiatrist because this is a taboo – this 'label' can spoil the patient's chances of an arranged marriage. If it is essential, then strict confidentiality should be maintained, even from the rest of his family.

Treatment can be considered under two headings, with due respect for religious principles.

Prevention. Pilgrimage to Mecca, *Haj*, during one's lifetime is one of the five fundamental principles of Islam. Muslim patients will need the appropriate immunisations, which should be anticipated by the GP.

Drug therapy. Every GP should be aware of the three major taboos in Islam which will affect drug treatment in the UK – alcohol, pork and non-Halal meat (ritually slaughtered).

Alcohol is forbidden because it impairs one's judgement. The pig is the only animal which lives in a sty, in which it happily eats, excretes and sleeps. In Islam, cleanliness is next to godliness. Symbolism forms the basis of a religious philosophy. Moreover, it is believed that one is what one eats, hence this stong taboo on pork.

Halal meat is the result of the ritual quick and painless killing of an animal. The blood is drained from the animal before it is dead. Therefore, Halal meat is considered to be infection-free and, because an animal's soul is believed to be in the blood, it is also believed to be soul-free.

These taboos give rise to two clinical problems. First, when a GP inadvertently prescribes a medication containing alcohol, and secondly, when he has to prescribe insulin.

Alcohol-containing medication. It is not uncommon for a devout Muslim to refuse conventional medicine, particularly in the month of Ramadan and near the time of his death, openly saying that 'English medicine contains alcohol'.

An English GP will never knowingly prescribe alcohol to a Muslim patient. However, there are many preparations commonly in use which contain alcohol and a GP may not be aware of this (see Table 2).

Insulin therapy. All non-synthetic insulins are either of pork or beef origin. Synthetic insulin is called human insulin, which is confusing to a Muslim patient because it sounds as if it is derived from human flesh, as mentioned elsewhere.

Pork insulin will not be accepted by a Muslim patient, and a Muslim would be horrified if he discovered that beef insulin was derived from non-Halal meat.

I suggest that beef insulin is prescribed and not pork, but a GP should be aware of the need to counsel the patient. If human insulin is to be used, the GP should volunteer to reassure his patient actively that this is *synthetic* insulin and is not made from human flesh. Human insulin is of pork origin and should be avoided. In the event of a patient being allergic to beef and human insulin, supportive counselling should be given to prepare him to accept the pork insulin as a life-saving decision.

Table 2 Alcohol-containing medications

Product	Alcohol	Amount
Tonics and nutrients		
Glycola	Alcohol 95%	0.5 ml/5 ml
Labiton	Alcohol	2.78 ml/10 ml
Multibionta	Pantothenyl alcohol	25 mg/10 ml
Neurophosphates	Ethanol	5.0% V/V
Parentrovite IMHP	Alcohol (No 1 amp)	140 mg/5 ml
Parentrovite IMM	Alcohol (No 1 amp)	80 mg/5 ml
Parentrovite IVHP	NONE	
Verdivitan	Alcohol	17% by volume
Antitussives		
Eumydrin	Ethyl alcohol	not known
Organidin	Alcohol 96%	1.25 ml/5 ml
Pavacol-D	Alcohol	not known
Triogesic elixir	Ethanol 96%	0.5 ml/5 ml
Triogesic tablets	NONE	
Eye preparations		
Hypotears	Polyvinyl alcohol	1%
Liquifilm	Polyvinyl alcohol	1.4%
Sno Tears	Polyvinyl alcohol	1.4%
Rectal applications		
Colifoam	Ethoxylated stearyl-alcohol	not known
	Cetyl alcohol	
Epifoam	Ethoxylated stearyl-alcohol	not known
	Cetyl alcohol	
Proctofoam HC	Ethoxylated stearyl alcohol	not known
	Cetyl alcohol	
Surgical and ENT		
Merocet solution	Alcoholic solution	not known
Merocet lozenges	NONE	
STD injection	Benzyl alcohol	2%
Surgical spirit	Alcohol	70%
Local application		
Alcoderm	Cetyl alcohol	not known
	Stearyl alcohol	not known
Alphosyl preparations	Refined alcoholic extract	5%
	of coal tar	
Betadine solution and paint	Alcoholic solution	not known
Betadine spray, gargle,		
mouthwash, ointment, scalp		
application, skin cleanser	NONE	
Betnovate scalp application	In alcoholic solution	not known
Betnovate lotion, ointment, cream	NONE	
Ceanel concentrate	Phenylethyl alcohol	7.5%
Diprobase cream	Cetostearyl alcohol	7.2%
Diprobase ointment	NONE	
Ionax scrub	Alcohol	not known
Ionil T shampoo	Hydro-alcoholic base	not known

(continued on next page)

Table 2 (continued)

Product	Alcohol	Amount
Locoid scalp application	In alcoholic solution	not known
Locoid cream, ointment	NONE	
Masse cream	Cetyl alcohol	2%
Metosyn scalp application	In alcohol solution	not known
Metosyn cream, ointment	NONE	
Oilatum emollient	Acetylated wool alcohol	5%
Oilatum cream	NONE	
Panoxyl gel	h-m-c-ethyl alcohol	not known
Polytar liquid	Oleyl alcohol	1%
Polytar Plus	Oleyl alcohol	1%
Pragmaton	Cetyl alcohol – coal	
	tar distillate	4%
Psorigel	Alcohol	33%
Spectraban	Alcoholic solution	not known
Sprilon aerosol	Wood alcohol	not known
	Cetyl alcohol	not known
Stie-Lasan	Cetyl alcohol	not known
Sudacrem	Benzyl alcohol	0.39%
Tarcortin	Refined alcoholic extract	
	of coal tar	5%
Tetmosol solution	alcoholic solution	not known
Tetmosol soap	NONE	
Ultrabase	Stearyl alcohol	8%
Unguentum	Cetostearyl alcohol	9%

Sources: MIMS, June, 1984; ABPI Data Sheet Compendium 1984/85; Medical Annual 1984

CHAPTER 24

NUTRITIONAL PROBLEMS IN ETHNIC GROUPS

General practitioners believe in food for thought, but the success of a general practice educational meeting could be indirectly related to the quality of gourmet food provided by the host agency! Everyone eats to live but some people live to eat. A balanced diet is vital for good health, but eating in excess is fraught with problems. English general practitioners tend to regard everyone as English and therefore to assume that every patient they see must be eating English food. Would it were as simple as this! In fact, there are English people who eat other ethnic foods, and ethnic minorities who eat English food as well as their traditional dishes – some eat more English food than the English do, and the unwary general practitioner can fall into a diagnostic trap. There are also large minorities who come from Commonwealth countries who eat their own cultural food, and although this has some benefits (see Chapter 6) it can produce clinical problems (Table 1), which affect local disease prevalence, consultation and prescribing.

Medical diets

Nutrition has always been a part of healing, and patients from ethnic minorities will not accept modern medicine unless practitioners take into account the nutritional implications of their diseases. Unfortunately this is not always the case and what happens is that the patient, having received medical advice from his doctor, then goes to his local pharmacist or a practitioner of alternative medicine for advice about his diet. Although most hospitals have dieticians, most general practices do not. General practitioners would do well to try to fill this gap, especially if they see patients from various ethnic groups.

A balanced diet is essential for well-being, but some ethnic minority patients on cult diets may suffer malnutrition. This can be avoided by offering advice about supplementing the diet with vitamins and minerals. Diseases that are induced by food include allergy, cancer, anaemia, heart disease, migraine and peptic ulcer. Other diseases related to food are obesity, diabetes mellitus, and constipation.

First published in *1986 RCGP Members' Reference Book*, 1986, pp.269–275 (Royal College of General Practitioners)

Table 1 Ethnic dietary problems

Diet	Content	Benefit	Problem
English	Low fibre	No breath smell	Constipation
Indian	Highly spiced	Cheap	Griping
Chinese	High fibre	Very light	Short stature
Vegetarian	High fibre	Very light	Anaemia
Vegan	No eggs	Frequent motions	Less food or drug absorption
Greek	Excess olive oil	Loose motions	Less food or drug absorption
Italian	High fat and pasta	Sustained release of energy (athletes' diet)	Obesity

There are 15 medical diets most commonly used for their therapeutic value: semi-liquid and low roughage (for the seriously ill), light and bland (for peptic ulcer), high roughage (constipation), low roughage (diarrhoea), low calorie (obesity), low carbohydrate – measured or selective (diabetes mellitus), low sodium and low calorie (cardiac failure), low sodium (oedema), low fat and high carbohydrate (liver disease), low cholesterol (hypercholesterolaemia), high protein and low fat (pancreatic disease), high protein and low sodium (nephrotic syndrome), low protein I (glomerulonephritis), low protein II (chronic renal failure), gluten free (coeliac disease) and low phenylalanine (phenylketonuria).

It is important to note in the first instance that all these suggestions are based on an English diet, and patients from other ethnic groups will need adjustments to their diet; for example, Chinese food has more fibre than English, and Indian food is very spicy. Secondly, ethnic minority patients have greater faith in a doctor who gives nutritional advice in conjunction with drug therapy. A Hakim, Vaid or other traditional healer in Eastern cultures always gives nutritional guidance along with pills or placebos.

Sometimes it is the omission, alteration or addition to certain foods that has the therapeutic effect and if the illness can be treated by diet alone, why resort to drug therapy? Nutrition plays a key role in the cause and treatment of an illness and if nutritional advice is given at the same time as medical advice, the result will be rewarding both for patient and practitioner. A general practitioner who shrugs his shoulders in answer to a query about food is in effect asking the patient to go away – and that patient will go straight to an alternative medicine practitioner.

Nutritional emergencies

Four foods can cause medical emergencies that, if not diagnosed promptly, may be fatal: ackee, karela, vetsin and yeast. Some English patients may also enjoy eating such foods.

Ethnic Jamaicans

Ackee is a fruit eaten as a native delicacy of Jamaica. Tinned ackee is available in the UK. Three-quarters of the West Indians in Britain come from Jamaica and visit their country of origin in holidays. They are very likely to bring back this fruit. When it is ripe and well cooked it makes a delicious dish. If unripe fruit is cooked, it is so poisonous that it can kill. Therefore children are not allowed near its forbidden plants. Ironically it resembles an apple.

Bush tea is also prepared from ackee, and its poison effect is known as Jamaican vomiting sickness. Two glycaemic factors are responsible for this food poisoning: hypoglycin A and hypoglycin B. This hypoglycaemia is more serious in those individuals who are undernourished[1]. It is the pod (the outer layer) and the film (which divides the fruit into two halves) that contain this poison (Table 2). I suggest that a general practitioner, especially one practising in an inner city area, should visit a local West Indian shop and familiarize himself with this fruit, usually in its tinned form. He may save a life as a result.

Table 2 Poisoning by the Jamaican fruit, ackee (hypoglycin A and B)

Layer	Colour	Property
Pod	Red	Poisonous
Pulp	Yellow	Edible
Seed	Black	Neither
Film	Red	Poisonous

Ethnic Asians

Karela (*Mormordica charantia*), cooked in a curry, is a popular choice of vegetarian Hindus (Indians or Kenyan Asians). Indian cuisine is becoming increasingly popular among English people. Karela is a vegetable resembling a gherkin. It has strong hypoglycaemic properties[2]. It is a much more potent hypoglycaemic agent than garlic or onions and it is customary to cook karela with both of these. Hakims (Muslim healers) use karela powder to treat diabetes. It has been shown to produce a small but significant improvement in glucose tolerance in diabetics.

In mild cases a patient may come to the surgery complaining of feeling weak, and it is important to exclude anaemia and depression before embarking on investigations and treatment. Karela potentiates the action of oral hypo-glycaemics and can cause prolonged hypoglycaemia, resulting in fainting or coma. Therefore this possibility must be considered in the differential diagnosis of such an emergency.

Ethnic Chinese

Vetsin is an additive and a sauce used in Chinese food such as wonton soup. It contains monosodium glutamate and some people are allergic to it. It is responsible for the Chinese restaurant syndrome described by Dr K W Heaton in 1968. After eating a Chinese meal, a susceptible person may experience symptoms lasting 30–45 minutes. These may include strange behaviour, confusion, or ataxia[3]. A typical symptom complex includes facial pressure, chest pain and a burning sensation in the head and upper trunk. It may be accompanied by dizziness, headache, nausea and vomiting. The glutamate is supposed to be a centrally active neurotransmitter. This might explain the pattern of reaction reported in some cases.

Further studies suggest that foods such as spiced tomato juice, orange juice and chocolate-flavoured milk – drinks so popular among Americans – can induce effects similar to those ascribed to glutamate[4].

According to a survey in 1985 there are 100,000 Chinese in Britain, many of whom work in family-run Chinese restaurants. A British general practitioner should be aware of this possible emergency in those eating Chinese foods, although it must be emphasized that such emergencies occur only rarely and there is no need to be unduly wary of Chinese foods.

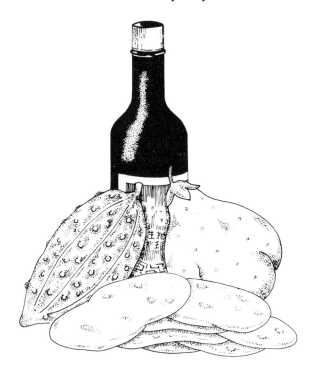

(Clockwise from top) Vetsin, ackee, nan, karela

Ethnic Afghans

Yeast is a kind of fungus that causes alcohol and carbon dioxide to be produced while it is developing. It is used to cause fermentation in wine- and beer-making, and as a raising agent in baking. It is not widely known that yeast in unlimited amounts is used as a raising agent when cooking nan bread. Nan is the main diet of Pathans coming from Afghanistan and Pakistan. Tandoori nan and chicken is an increasingly popular food among the English who frequent Indian restaurants. A similar bread called pitta is used by the Greeks and Cypriots. If a patient has to be on monoamine oxidase inhibitors, yeast is strongly contra-indicated to avoid a hypertensive crisis[5].

Not only is nan the main carbohydrate in these ethnic diets but also higher proportions of yeast may be used in some cases, depending on ethnic customs. There are two problems with this: first, an ethnic minority patient may not be aware that the unlimited amount of yeast in his daily diet is medically important unless the doctor tells him; and secondly, if a doctor tells him point blank to stop eating nan when on monoamine oxidase inhibitors the advice will fall on deaf ears unless the doctor suggests an alternative bread and spends some time counselling the patient. After all, having to give up one's traditional daily food is a major decision.

Problems with common food

The main carbohydrate in English food is potato, in African food, cassava, in Asian, chapati and in Chinese food, rice. When these carbohydrates are taken in excess they may lead to chronic diseases.

Ethnic English

The English eat more potato chips than other ethnic groups, but bread and sugar is consumed by all ethnic groups. The total requirement of carbohydrates per day is about 375g; the use of potatoes within this limit is justified, but exceeding this limit is a serious health hazard. Too much potato is as harmful as too much bread and sugar: potato storage is converted to glucose and any surplus glucose is converted to fat. Obesity and excess fat are associated with the risk of coronary heart disease, which is still the biggest killer disease in the UK. The excessive use of potatoes must be avoided.

Chicken and chips is a good meal but if it is taken every day to the exclusion of other main meals, it can lead to folic acid deficiency[6]. This is more common among elderly English men.

Ethnic Africans

Cassava (mohugo) is mainly taken by ethnic Africans but not West Indians, who eat rice (and peas). Cassava contains very small amounts of thiocyanates and, when eaten in excess over a long period, these can cause pancreatic diabetes.

Ethnic Asians

Chapatis (Asian unleavened bread) are exclusively eaten by Asian (Indians, Pakistanis, Bangladeshis and Sri Lankans). This is their main source of carbohydrates and is eaten in large amounts daily. Chapati flour contains phytic acid, which binds with calcium to make calcium phytate, which is excreted, thereby reducing the available calcium in the gut. The main function of Vitamin D is to promote calcium absorption through the calcium binding and transporting protein of the intestinal mucosa. This protein is not formed if there is a vitamin D deficiency. As a result of the daily chapati intake, insufficient calcium is absorbed despite the presence of adequate vitamin D.

Thus both vitamin D and calcium should be given to prevent or treat fetal or toddler's rickets and osteomalacia. The Asian population has the highest prevalence of rickets and osteomalacia of any group in the UK (Table 3).

Table 3 Nutritional deficiencies

Ethnic group	Subgroup	Deficiency	Reason
English	Elderly	Vitamin C (widower's scurvy) Folic acid	Tinned food. No fresh greens Mainly fish and chip diet
Irish	Men	All vitamins	Alcohol consumption
Asians	Women	Vitamin D (osteomalacia)	Chapati diet
	Children	(rickets)	Chapati diet
	Fetus	(rickets)	Chapati diet (mother)
	Gujaratis	Iron	Vegans or vegetarians
Africans	Rastafarians	Protein (kwashiorkor)	Cult diet

Exposure to sunlight is equal in all ethnic groups in this country. Clothing varies according to climate and even Muslims who observe purdah go out shopping and make good use of their sun lounges. If the colour of the skin was the criterion for the aetiology, Afro-Caribbeans would have a far higher incidence of rickets, but this is not the case. Asian general practitioners often give courses of calcium preparations to ethnic Asian patients, especially women, to the surprise of the manufacturers. I suggest that rickets and osteomalacia may not only be vitamin D deficiency diseases but may also be accompanied by calcium deficiency diseases, and the evidence leans so heavily towards chapati phytic acid that more research is needed in this area.

Phytates are known to reduce not only the bioavailability of calcium but also that of iron and zinc. A very high intake of phytates is clearly undesirable in infants, children, pregnant or lactating women, and possibly the elderly[7]. It is inconceivable that any Asian will stop eating chapatis but it cannot be overemphasized that a British general practitioner should look for these deficiency diseases and should consider prescribing calcium along with vitamin D as a therapeutic or preventive measure in this ethnic group.

Ethnic Chinese

Rice is the main carbohydrate in Chinese food. For reasons yet to be discovered, this may cause post-bulbar duodenal ulcers[8]. Other rice-eating ethnic minority groups are West Indians, Bangladeshis and South Indians. A posterior duodenal ulcer carries a risk of secondary haemorrhage by erosion of a large vessel. An early referral to a consultant surgeon could be very rewarding for diagnosis and management.

Conclusion

British general practitioners should realize that there are now many ethnic minority groups in Britain and they should be prepared to care for all of them. However, they should appreciate that all ethnic groups are different. They do not all eat the same food and a general practitioner should be aware of the various ethnic diets.

Ethnic diets can both cause and cure nutritional problems. A nutritional history should always be taken and a clinical examination may reveal signs of nutritional excess or deficiency. Nutritional aspects should also be considered during investigation, consultation and prescribing.

If these guidelines are followed, patients will be well served and will not need to consult other health professionals or healers, as they sometimes do now.

References

1. Donaldson, D. (1984). Causes and mechanisms of hypoglycaemia. *Faculty News*, **4**, 5–6
2. Leatherdale, B.A., Panesar, R.K. and Singh, G. *et al.* (1981). Improvement in glucose tolerance due to *Mormodica charantia* (karela). *Br. Med. J.*, **1**, 3
3. Editorial (1984). *Journal of the American Medical Association*, **252**, 899
4. Ebert, A.G. (1984). Chinese restaurant syndrome. *Br. Med. J.*, **289**, 1626
5. Dally, P.J. (1978). Drug therapy. In: Connolly, J. (ed.) *Therapy Options in Psychiatry*. London, Pitman Medical
6. Dickerson, J.W.T. (1984). Patients in the community prone to dietary deficiencies. *Faculty News*, **4**, 1–2
7. Southgate, D. (1985). Dietary fibre. *Fit for Future (Farleycare Journal)*, **1**, 3
8. Craig, O. (1978). Barium meal X-rays of the gut. Tutorial at the Royal College of Surgeons. Unpublished

NUTRITION AND MULTI-ETHNIC GROUPS

SUMMARY

Growth and health depend on food. You are what you eat. Cultural eating habits are based on low cost and availability of a food in the local market. Religious restrictions on a particular food are meant to prevent moral, psychological and physical harm. In English food; excessive use of chips may lead to obesity and heart disease. Low fibre with high fat may contribute to cancer of the colon. Bangladeshi rice eaters may develop post-bulbar duodenal ulcer. Japanese raw fish diet may predispose to cancer of the stomach. Asian chapati diet may cause rickets and osteomalasia. Vegetarians may get iron deficiency anaemia. An Indian vegetable 'karela' in a curry may potentiate the action of chlorpropamide (diabenase) and lead to prolonged hypoglycaemia resulting in fainting or coma. A Jamaican native dish of the delicacy 'ackee' if cooked unripe can kill.

This section deals with such clinical points for a busy doctor and practical tips for other health workers who care for multi-ethnic groups in the UK.

MULTI-ETHNIC GROUPS

Morphologically, the world population can be divided into four multi-ethnic groups. There are many subgroups and, using the criteria of bone structure and skin complexion, we can differentiate the following groups:

1. Europeans; white (pink)
2. Asians; brown (light-skinned)
3. Africans; black
4. Chinese; yellow (fair)

The bone structure, especially facial features, is similar in Europeans and Asians.

MULTI-ETHNIC GROUPS IN THE UK

Migration is mainly occupational. Big industrial cities have attracted the English from rural areas and ethnic minority groups from Ireland and overseas countries. The ethnic minority groups include the Irish, Asians, West Indians, Chinese, Greeks, Italians, Spanish and Cypriots. These groups are mainly employed by: (1) National Health Service (2) building industry (3) factories (4) British rail and London transport (5) catering.

The self-employed have opened restaurants and small businesses. Women outworkers and moonlighters as well as the self-employed eat at irregular intervals because they have to work long and unsocial hours.

First published in *J. Roy. Soc. Health*, **101**, No.5, Oct. 1981, pp.187–195 (Royal Society of Health)

DIET AND SOCIAL CLASS

A rich man eats what he likes – a poor man eats what he gets. The social class system in the UK and the caste system in India are based on the father's occupation. The choice of food varies with the income of a family.

Social classes (official)

I.   Professional – clergyman, doctors, directors, lawyers
II.   Intermediate – farmers, teachers, nurses, civil servants
III.   Skilled – clerks, typists, shop assistants, miners and skilled industrial workers
IV.   Semi-skilled – agricultural and other semi-skilled workers
V.   Unskilled – building and dock workers, labourers, cleaners

Castes (semi-official)

I.   Brahmins – high priests and the highest caste people
II.   Kshtriya – armed forces and civil servants
III.   Vaishya – business people
IV.   Kshudra – untouchables; cleaners

Communists (unofficial)

I.   Communist farmers
II.   Clergymen
III.   Non-Communists and dissidents

As a person's occupation may change, his diet may alter but dietary habits may remain unchanged.

VARIOUS DIETS

A.   Omnivorous – (lean meat) most of the world population
B.   Vegetarians – (eggs and milk included) Hindus especially Gujarati Indians
C.   Vegans – (eggs and milk excluded) – some Hindus
D.   Special
       (1)   No pork – Religions (Halal meat or Kosher meat) – Muslims (Arabs and Pakistanis), Jews (Israelis)
       (2)   No beef – Hindus (Indians)
       (3)   Fruitarian – (fruit only) – some vegans
       (4)   Zen Macrobiotics – (whole grain cereals e.g. brown rice) – Chinese and Japanese
       (5)   Health foods – (soya beans products + vitamins and honey) – therapeutic and preventive

(6) Slimming diets
    (i)   Low energy diet (1000 calories) – therapeutic and preventive
    (ii)   High protein, high fat diet
(7) Fasting – Religious – Muslims (Arabs and Pakistanis) one month in the year – Ramadan

Favourite diets in the UK

English: potatoes, fish, chicken, pork and lamb
Americans: steaks and hamburgers
Italian; pizza and spaghettis, high fat, fish, pasta
Greek: kebabs, rice and nan
West Indian; pork, chicken and rice
Indian: a)   North – meat and wheat (curry and chapati)
           b)   South – fish and rice
           c)   Gujarati – vegetarians and vegans
Pakistani; meat and wheat (tandoori meat, chapati and nan)
Bangladeshi: fish and rice
Chinese: fish, rice and vegetables

DIETARY HABITS

Eating habits

a)   Knife and fork: Europeans. Advantage – it reduces the risk of food poisoning, dysentry or indigestion.
b)   Clean hands: Asians. Advantage – one rinses mouth after every meal along with washing hands. So it reduces the risk of dental decay due to food particles.
c)   Chop sticks: Chinese. Advantage – one takes one's time eating.

Toilet habits

European: high seat and toilet paper. The job is not done until paper work is finished.
Asian: low seat and water wash. This prevents piles, which is one of the three commonest causes of iron deficiency anaemia in the UK (others being peptic ulcers and heavy periods).

Diet and occupations

In work places, especially factories, the dietary restriction e.g. pork, beef or all meat and dietary habits of eating with clean hands on the same table where the English workers are eating, may cause problems. The toilet habits, if not sympathetically tackled, may lead to sickness absence.

Diet and health services

There are specific problems in giving injections. Measles vaccine is prepared in egg medium. Insulins are prepared in pork or beef mediums. Vegetarians and Muslim and Hindu diabetics will run into difficulties.

DIET AND DISEASE

General concern

Height and weight

Vegetarians differ from omnivores in many respects. Their energy intake, height and weight are less and their stools are softer, but their capacity to do physical and mental work is the same as meat eaters. Mahatama Gandhi was a vegetarian. It is not surprising therefore when we find that the English height and weight chart (Tanner) does not apply to Gujarati hindu children who are vegetarians. The Chinese and Malaysians who consume less lean meat are smaller and lighter than Europeans, Africans and other Asians. Their normal babies are of light birthweight and are small.

Benefits of fibre

Dietary fibre is usually of plant origin. The vegetarian and Chinese diets have it in abundance. Wheatbran is most effective weight for weight. Bran breakfast cereals which are unrefined are probably the best. It should be taken in moderation. An excess of fibre can cause abdominal discomfort from colonic gas. The diseases which can be prevented by fibre include: constipation, diverticular disease, irritable bowel syndrome, anal fissure, gallstones, cancer of the colon, ulcerative colitis, hiatus hernia, haemorrhoids (piles), appendicitis and obesity.

Allergy

Asian healers such as Hakims and Vaids are aware of food allergies. In treating almost any disease avoidance of certain foods is advised. As a result an Asian patient will ask his doctor, 'What food should be avoided?'. This is called 'perhaiz'. The Asian baby is most liable to an intolerance to lactose, a sugar fraction of milk. This may result in diarrhoea and vomiting.

One can be allergic to any food but the common food allergens are in milk, egg, tea, coffee, chocolate, sugar, beef, wheat, corn, yeast, pork, fish, cheese, rice, alcohol. tomatoes, additives and preservatives, apples and peanuts. The first ten foods in this list are related to migraine. Food allergy may cause eczema, urticaria, migraine, asthma, rhinitis, joint pain, abdominal pain, diarrhoea, mouth ulcers, palpitations, anxiety, depression and behaviour problems.

'The exclusion diet' used in treatment of food allergy consists of lamb, pears and bottled spring water. These three foods are least likely to cause allergy. It appears that this problem of food allergy may have given birth to the varieties of accepted and bizarre diets.

Nutritional deficiencies

In vegetarians iron deficiency anaemia may occur. In unusual diets protein deficiency and vitamin deficiency diseases may occur. In the elderly who neglect their diet and do not take vegetables or fruits, scurvy – a vitamin C deficiency – is noted by general practitioners. The parents who put their children on unusual diets causing nutritional deficiencies are best dealt with as 'child abuse' cases. Rarely in the UK, cases of kwashiorkor and marasmus have occured in such families.

Mental illness and wheat

In schizophrenics, wheat antibodies have been found to be significantly higher and yeast antibodies lower than in the general population. The clinical value of these findings is under consideration. Some research workers believe that there might be a strong link between diet and depressive illness.

Salt intake and hypertension

Salt may play an important aetiological role in essential hypertension, at least in predisposed individuals. A salt-free diet (rice and fruits) undoubtedly proved effective before the days of antihypertensive drugs. However salt depletion is a side-effect of such a diet, especially in a patient with diarrhoea. Primitive cultures who live on vegetarian diets with low salt have less prevalence of hypertension. Studies in the USA show that ethnic Africans have a greater prevalence of hypertension, possibly because they have a greater sensitivity than Europeans to the hypertensive effects of sodium.

Nutritional factors in coronary heart disease

Coronary heart disease is called the modern epidemic in the Western world. It is the largest killer disease in the UK. It is becoming more common in ethnic Asians who have adopted the Western way of life. Middle-aged men aged 30 – 50 are at greatest risk of heart attack. But heart attacks are not necessarily fatal. Many people who suffer an attack recover, and by following their doctor's advice can continue to lead a normal life. The risk factors include the following:

(a) Obesity – the commonest nutritional disorder in Western society
(b) Diabetes – diet plays a part in its control
(c) Soft water – reason unknown but it may be due to less calcium and more toxic metals e.g. lead, calcium and mercury
(d) High intake of sugar, salt and animal fat
(e) Low content of dietary fibre

Cancer

Recent evidence suggests that up to half of all cancers may be related to diet.

(a)   There is a strong association between total fat intake and the incidence of breast and colon cancer.
(b)   A small reduction of energy intake can dramatically reduce the total incidence of tumours in animals.
(c)   A lower intake of vitamin A is associated with lung, bladder, stomach and colorectal cancer.

Oral cancer, especially cancer of the cheek, is more common in Pakistanis and Indians. Studies on such patients in Pakistan and India show low concentrations of serum retinoids. Cancer of the cheek may be associated with a unique Asian habit of betel (pan) chewing. This delicacy is used by one tenth of the world population living in Asia and the Far East. Betel chewing consists of a mixture of betel leaf, tobacco, lime, katechu and betel nut. This mixture is kept for a long time in the mouth between gums and cheek. The chronic irritation may lead to cancer of the cheek.

American studies have shown that the following types of cancers have ethnic differences:

(a)   In ethnic Africans – 50% more common cancers are: oesophagus, multiple myloma, cervix, vagina, penis, prostate, liver, stomach.
(b)   In ethnic Europeans – 50% more common cancers are: lips, malignant melanoma, testicles, eyes, thyroid, bladder, uterus, brain, lymphoma.

All these cancers except thyroid, bladder and uterus have racial factors in their aetiology, although what these factors are is still unknown. Possibly genetic as well as environmental factors including diet are important variables.

Special concern

Europeans

1.   Alcoholism
     Alcoholism is the fifth common cause of death in the UK. An alcoholic risks an accident, divorce and the sack. "Alcohol provokes the desire but takes away the performance" (Shakespeare). It is less common in the Eastern society and almost non-existent publicly in the Muslim countries.

2.   Obesity
     The most common nutritional disorder in Western society is obesity which is mainly due to excessive use of potatoes in the English diet and pizza + spaghetti in the Italian diet. In developing countries hunger is a common problem. That is why the advertisements in the West carry sex appeal while in the East they consist of food appeal.

3.   Dental diseases
     Excessive use of sticky sweets, chocolates and sugar, leads to dental
     diseases.

Asians (Pakistanis and Indians)

1.   Rickets and osteomalacia
     A chapati diet is exclusive to Asian people. A child is introduced to it at the
     age of four months. Chapati flour contains phytic acid which combines with
     dietary calcium to make calcium phytate which is then excreted. Rickets is
     more common in ethnic Asian children age 1–4 years, than in ethnic
     Africans or ethnic Europeans, for this reason.

2.   TB glands, typhoid and dysentry
     These diseases are acquired from infected milk and water. Travellers to the
     Asian subcontinent may suffer from these diseases.

3.   Karela
     Karela is a popular choice of vegetarian Hindus (Indians). It is cooked in a
     curry. This vegetable has a hypoglycaemic effect. It was used in place of
     insulin in old Indian therapies. It can potentiate the action of chlorprop-
     amide (Diabenese) and cause prolonged hypoglycaemia resulting in
     fainting or coma. Sometimes non-vegetarians also eat karela curry.

Bangladeshis and Chinese

These are rice and fish eating populations. Recent studies suggest that
'post-bulbar duodenal ulcer' is more common in rice eating populations. West
Indians also consume rice as their main diet.

Japanese

The incidence of stomach cancer is very high in the Japanese. It is suggested
to be due to eating raw fish.

West Indians

Three-quarters of West Indians in the UK are Jamaicans. 'Ackee' is a
vegetable eaten as a native delicacy in Jamaica. If picked from plants unripe
and cooked, it can kill. Therefore children are not allowed near this forbidden
vegetable. When it is ripe and cooked well, it is delicious.

Hot spicy food especially containing red chillis is a gastric and colonic irritant. To
avoid heartburn, abdominal discomfort due to gas and loose motions, one
should use yoghurt with Indian and West Indian foods.

CONCLUSIONS

Today's world has become a global village. Recent research has shown that diet has a direct influence on health, disease and its management. It varies between different ethnic groups. A greater understanding and an effort to improve nutrition will promote health.

Further reading

Albert, M.J. *et al.* (1980). Vegetarian immigrants may lack vitamin B. *Doctor*, 20th March, 27

Arnold, K. (1980). Gastrointestinal diseases; the benefits of fibre. *Geriatric Medicine*, November 60–67

Brandon, L. (1980). Ackee dishes – ackee souffle, ackee and cheese filling, ackee rice and cheese, ackee served as first course. *A Merry Go Round of Recipes from Jamaica*, 46–48

Brook, O. (1981). Vitamin D supplements in pregnancy. *J. Maternal Child Health*, January, 18–20

Burnan, D. (1979). Adolescent nutrition. *The Practitioner*, **222**, 615–623

Craig, O. (1978). Barium meal X-rays of the gut. Tutorial at the Royal College of Surgeons of England. (unpublished)

Dickerson, J.W.T. (1980). Nutrition in cancer patients. *Doctor*, 3rd April, 22: Nutrition in an age of technology, University of Surrey University Lecture (1980)

Dickerson, J.W.T. and Fehily, A.M. (1979). Bizarre and unusual diets. *The Practitioner*, **222**, 643–647

Dillon, M.J. (1979). Malnutrition in infants receiving cult diets; a form of child abuse. *Br. Med. J.*, 1st February, 296–298

Dunnigan, M.G. *et al.* (1980). Policy of prevention of Asian rickets in Britain. *Br. Med. J.*, **282**, 357–360

Eagle, R. (1980). Your friendly neighbourhood hakim. *World Medicine*, July, 19–22

Editorial (1980). Indo-Chinese refugees in Britain. *Br. Med. J.*, May, 1274

Ellis, H. (1977). Carcinoma of the stomach. In: *Lecture Notes on General Surgery*, p.183

Forrest, D. (1980). Feeding practices in the Asian community. *MIMS Magazine*, December, 21–29

Goodwig, G. (1980). The problems of Vietnamese children in Britain. *J. Maternal and Child Health*, August, 307–312

Kenny, R.A. (1979). Possible psychiatric reactions to monosodium glutamate. *N. Engl. J. Med.*, **300**, 503

Kenny, R.A. (1980). Chinese Restaurant Syndrome. *The Lancet*, 9th February, 311–312

Kirton, V. (1980). *Allergy* published by Allergy Information Centre. *How to Cope with Food Allergies* published by Allergy Information Centre

Leffal, L.D. (1980). Cancer types in ethnic groups. Clinical News. *Doctor*, 22

Levin, B. and Harowitz, D. (1979). Dietary fibre. *Med. Clin. N. Am.*, **63**, September, 1043–1053. Abstract in *Medical Digest*, November, 32–34

Lobo, E.H. (1978). *Children of Immigrants to Britain*, Hodder and Stoughton

MacCormich, C. (1980). Health care problems in ethnic minority groups. *MIMS Magazine*, July, 33–40

Maclean, U. (1980). Women and family health. *MIMS Magazine*, August, 31–37

Mann, G.V. (1980). Food intake and resistance to disease. *The Lancet*, 7th June, 1218

Marino, D.D. and King, O.C. (1980). Nutritional concerns during adolescence. *Paediatr. Clin. N. Am.*, 27th February, 125–139. Abstract in *Medical Digest*, November 1980, 38–41

Monro, J. (1980). Seeking links between diet and mental health. *Doctor*, 11th December, 27

Monro, J. *et al.* (1980). Food allergy in migraine. *The Lancet*, July, 1–3

Phillips, S.J. and Pearson, R.J. (1981). Dealing with Vietnamese refugees (Practice Observed). *Br. Med. J.*, **282**, 525–527

Phillips. S.J. (1980). Vietnamese refugees. *J. Maternal Child Health*, November, 442-443

Politt, N.T. (1980). Clinical osteomalacia in settlers to England. *Doctor*, May, 20

Ragaveer-Saran, M.K. and Keddle, N.C. (1980). Drop in Appendicitis. *Br. J. Surg.*, **67**, 681. Due to high fibre diet? *Medical News*, November, 12

Scott, P.P. (1979). Food additives and contaminants. *The Practitioner*, **222**, 648–655

Spilsbury, S. (1981). Catering for ethnic minorities. *Hosp. Health Serv. Purchasing*, February, 48

Turner, G.W.D. (1979). Fat and coronary heart disease. *The Practitioner*, **222**, 601–610

Warmer, J. (1980). Food intolerance in infants and toddlers. *MIMS Magazine*, 15th December, 37–45

Werther, J.L. (1980). Breast cancer and fat consumption. *NY State J. Med.*, **80**, 1401

Wraith, D.G. (1980). Food allergies – the allergies in general practice. A reprint for *Modern Medicine*

Yudkin, J. *et al.* (1980). Effects of high dietary sugar. *Br. Med. J.*, **281**, 22nd November, 1396

Dear Sir

Nutrition and multi-ethnic groups

I would be grateful for an opportunity to comment on the article 'Nutrition and multi-ethnic groups' by Dr B.A. Qureshi in the October 1981 issue of the Royal Society of Health Journal.

'The most common nutritional disorder in Western Society is obesity which is mainly due to excessive use of potatoes in the English diet.' This is rather a surprising statement as it has been suggested many times that the consumption of potatoes should be increased[1–3]. It is also worth noting that, in 1979, potatoes accounted for only 5% of the total calorie intake in the UK as well as making a significant contribution to the total intakes of iron (almost 7%), thiamin (approx. 10%), nicotinic acid (approx. 10%) and vitamin C (24%)[4].

'In English food; excessive use of chips may lead to obesity and heart disesase.' Excessive use of many foods can lead to problems. Why pick on chips? They are consumed in fairly large quantities by some people in the UK, but to what extent should this be discouraged? The main objection to chips seems to be the fat content and there are two points to bear in mind. The first is that chips are rarely fried in animal fat. The second point is that the fat content of chips can vary a great deal. In fact the fat can provide from 28 to 48% of the total calories in chips (calculated from data in reference 5). Surely a food which makes a significant contribution to the total diet and has a fat content which provides 28% of its calories is not to be discouraged. In this case it might be more profitable to encourage people to look critically at their methods of preparation rather than ask them to change their dietary habits.

One final comment. If a reduction in calorie intake is desirable then a reduction in the consumption of sugar and/or alcohol might be a better way of achieving this.

Yours faithfully

A Lecturer in Food and Nutrition

References

1. DHSS (1978) *Eating for Health*. HMSO, London
2. Passmore, R., Hollingsworth, D.F. and Robertson, J. (1979). *Br. Med. J.*, **280**, 527
3. McLaren, D. (1981). *The 1980 Nutrition Award Prize-winning Papers*. Van den Berghs and Jurgens Ltd
4. MAFF (1981). *Household Food Consumption and Expenditure: 1979*. HMSO, London
5. Paul, A.A. and Southgate, D.A.T. (1978). *McCance and Widdowson's The Composition of Foods*, 4th Edn. HMSO, London

Dr Bashir Qureshi has replied:

Mr Hogarth's letter contains extremely valuable information and I wish that I could totally agree with him. Current scientific evidence suggests that an excess of potato is as harmful as bread or sugar: the potato starch is converted into glucose, the surplus glucose is converted into fat, the excess of fat is associated with a risk of coronary heart disease, which is the biggest killer disease in the UK, especially in middle-aged European men, who are most needed by their families.

Multi-ethnic observations reveal that the bread and sugar is consumed by all ethnic groups but the English eat more potato chips than ethnic Asians, African and Chinese workers in the UK.

Daily total requirements for carbohydrates is about 375 grams. The use of potato within this limit is justified but exceeding this limit has serious health hazards and must be discouraged. Strong views should not colour the real news.

Dr Bashir Qureshi

CHAPTER 25

SKIN PROBLEMS ENCOUNTERED IN MULTI-ETHNIC PATIENTS

Transcultural medicine involves the clinical and consultant encounters between a doctor of one ethnic and a patient of another. In addition to the medical aspects (physical, psychological and social), it is necessary to consider the problems which may arise because of the ethnic differences, and necessary to consider communication, religion, culture and ethnicity.

A British GP spends a lot of his consultation time dealing with chronic skin conditions. While an English patient (more informed by the media in his own language) accepts that there is no permanent cure for many such illnesses and is happy to discuss the progress with his GP and to comply with that GP's treatment and an occasional referral to a consultant dermatologist, most ethnic minority patients have different expectations. Such a patient is very alarmed by the appearance of a skin disease, worries that it could be infectious, dreads its cultural consequences, attributes it to sins committed in this or a previous life, and expects a miraculous, permanent cure. If the GP does not understand his inner feelings the patient will demand to see the top consultant dermatologist, and on the quiet will consult with private practitioners, particularly alternative therapists. Much time, money and suffering can therefore be spared by a successful GP consultation.

This chapter highlights some practical points to further transcultural understanding in such consultations, whether in the GP's surgery or in a dermatological outpatient clinic.

COMMUNICATION BARRIERS

Although skin disease carries some stigma in British society, in ethnic minority cultures dermatological problems produce great distress, and this fact should be clearly understood from the outset.

Social outcast. An English patient will happily discuss his or her skin condition with the next-door neighbour or in the GP's waiting room. A patient from an eastern culture will conceal it from everyone including his family and, in an attempt to avoid the curiosity of any neighbours attending the surgery, will arrive at the end of the surgery time – an act considered unforgiveable in the eyes of a GP's receptionist!

First published in *Dermatology in Practice*, **4**(4), August 1986, pp.11 – 16 (Medical Tribune Group)

In eastern cultures a skin disease carries a stigma because of long-standing memories of widespread leprosy and the fear of contagion. In medieval times there was no adequate treatment for acute or chronic skin conditions and obviously the appearance of such an illness was considered so sinister that the victim was shunned by everybody. Cultural beliefs are very deeprooted and even now, in spite of westernisation, such a patient feels deeply ashamed. A receptionist should not frown upon such a patient as it will make him feel even worse, and a GP should be more sympathetic and reassure the patient about the nature of his condition – explanation rather than discussion is called for in this situation.

Beat the queue. As with committees and time-keeping, religiously forming a queue is a unique British habit. Germans and Asians are not queue-conscious, and this will not only annoy the overworked receptionist but will also infuriate the English patients who have been patiently awaiting their turn. In such a situation the receptionist should politely tell the ethnic minority patient to observe the queue, which he will be happy to do. Similarly, he may not be punctual for an appointment at the skin clinic or may not even ring to cancel, simply not turning up, because he is unaware of the seriousness of this omission. Worse still, he may turn up without an appointment and expect to be seen! However, if politely asked to keep the appointment at the right time by the receptionist or the doctor he will willingly comply. There is no need for anyone to feel annoyed.

Another avoidable cultural encounter is related to smell. The English do not like the smell of curry on clothing. Muslims abhor the smell of alcohol on the breath, and Sikhs hate smoking. Such patients will go to great lengths to avoid waiting in the same room, resulting in cultural misunderstanding. This problem could be avoided by positive health education.

RELIGIOUS MATTERS

A British GP believes that he must offer care to a defined population, irrespective of race, religion and social class. In nearly all consultations the patient differ in some way from the doctor; sometimes this difference produces difficulties. Usually a British doctor is a Protestant with liberal views, but an ethnic minority patient is likely to be of a different religion. He may be a Catholic, Hindu, Muslim, Sikh, Jew or Buddhist, and to him, religion is all important. No doctor can succeed in a consultation and ensure compliance in a multi-ethnic setting without due regard to religion, ethnicity and the socio-economic considerations of the patient. A positive approach in this matter is mandatory.

Myths and superstitions. A Hindu believes in astrology and it is not uncommon for such a patient to tell the GP: 'I was destined to have eczema because that is what my stars foretold'. Hindus believe in re-incarnation and some believe that skin disease is the result of their sins in an earlier life. They may have a very fatalistic attitude and consider the GP's role to be merely supplementary.

Muslims think that skin diseases are sometimes manifestations of God's punishment for sins committed in this life, and may turn to prayer and the religious sacrifice of a lamb or a cockerel, killed in a ritual slaughter and distributed to the poor. They may decide to visit holy shrines and be given charms by faith healers to wear around the arm or neck. They may also consider the GP's treatment to be supplementary because they believe that such treatment will only work if it is the will of Allah.

In Asian, Chinese, south-east Asian and Afro-Caribbean cultures influenced by various religions there is a common belief that a stranger might have cast an 'evil eye' on the person so inflicting skin disease, or that a wicked neighbour or relative may be using black magic to the same effect. Such people also believe that a patient with a skin disease must have broken a religious taboo and annoyed his ancestors, the gods or saints. A British GP might dismiss this idea very lightly, causing the ethnic minority patient to lose faith in him and turn to alternative medicine. I would suggest that the GP has a counseling session to give the patient a rational explanation, thereby reaching a compromise.

Sometimes an Asian patient is sent abroad to visit a holy spa or river for the treatment of skin disease. It is said that these waters contain minerals and medicinal compounds. Since the lifespan of certain skin diseases such as eczema are naturally self-limiting, is it realistic to attribute the natural recovery to this ritualistic treatment?

Alcohol-containing applications. Alcohol is taboo in Islam and no devout Muslim will ever use an application which contains alcohol. Because of mutual politeness neither the British GP nor his Muslim patient will refer to this point, and the GP's prescription will remain untouched and the condition will get worse, despite the so-called 'treatment'. A complete list of alcohol-containing products as listed in *MIMS* and the *Data Sheet Compendium* has been published (see Chapter 23).

Religious rituals. Shaving the head of an infant before naming it is a ritual practised by Muslims, Hindus and Sikhs. Head-shaving is also a religious custom of Muslims on a pilgrimage, Hindus visiting holy shrines, and Buddhist monks. Conversely, long hair and beards are traditions of many religions, though only Sikh men are not allowed to cut their hair at all, and keep it tidy with a comb worn under the turban. Hindus may have a tuft of long hair at the back of a shaved scalp (for example, the Hari Krishna cult).

In this respect there are two things which a GP or skin specialist should bear in mind: first, a patient may be too busy praying and working to wash his long hair often enough, this applying particularly to a schoolchild who may develop skin conditions including pediculosis. Second, head-shaving rituals are performed by religious practitioners who are not trained barbers, as is the case during Haj (pilgrimage to Mecca) and as a result there could be multiple scarring. The GP should not be afraid to ask the reason behind such scars.

Moharram scars are caused by the ritual self-beating of the chest and back with hands, knives and chains, carried out by devout Shia Muslims from Iran and Lebanon in the annual mourning ceremony commemorating the brutal killing of the Imam Hussein and Hassan, the grandsons of the Prophet Muhammed, in AD631, in Koofa (Iraq). These scars should not be mistaken for child abuse or dermatitis artefacta, and treatment, if required, should be offered sympathetically.

ETHNIC DIFFERENCES

A British GP or skin specialist is highly trained in basic dermatology; this section will be confined therefore to those aspects of skin disease which reflect true ethnic differences (Table 1).

Ethnic English. As with freckles, red hair and varicose veins, strawberry marks (in children) are more common in this ethnic group. An English mother will always be conscious of the risk of a mole becoming malignant, and needs reassurance from her doctor that such moles constitute a benign condition. Occasionally the condition may be seen in a light-skinned Asian child, and must not be mistaken for a cigarette burn.

Table 1   Skin disease patterns in ethnic groups

Ethnic group	Common diseases
English	Strawberry mark Basal cell carcinoma (rodent ulcer) Industrial dermatitis Psoriasis Varicose ulcers Tattoos
Asian	Pityriasis alba Mongolian spots Chloasma Dark rings around the eyes Tikka or sari metal-thread dermatitis Ankle eczema (neurodermatitis) Hirsuties Lupus vulgaris Vaccination scars Smallpox scars Ear and nose piercing
Afro-Caribbean	Keloid scars Ceremonial scars (Africans) Traction alopecia Pityriasis nigra Pomade acne
Chinese	Port wine stains Fungal infections between fingers and toes Hydration acne (humid environment in restaurants)
Gujaratis (India, Kenya, Uganda)	Swastika tattoos
Iranians	Moharram scars

Ethnic Asians. Some skin conditions are commonly seen much more in Asian concern and dark rings around the eyes. Both conditions cause great to the patient and relatives because they fear that they will have a detrimental effect on an arranged marriage.

Pityriasis alba causes great confusion. It consists of hypopigmented patches appearing mainly on the face (generally during the summer months) and occurs predominantly in schoolchildren. Asian parents mistake this for vitiligo or nutritional deficiencies. They panic and bring the child to the GP demanding urgent referral to a dermatologist, hoping for an instant cure. School teachers mistake these patches for ringworm infestation and try to exclude the child from school. Although it is thought to be a form of atopic eczema, it does not always respond to hydrocortisone ointments and thus causes additional distress to the parents. All that is needed is tactful handling by the GP, with reassurance to the school authorities that it is non-contagious and to the parents that it is a benign and self-limiting condition. The use of moisturisers and medicated bath oils by the affected individual may be helpful.

Ethnic Afro-Caribbeans. A keloid scar represents an exaggerated collagen response to skin injury. Afro-Caribbeans are predisposed to the development of keloid scars and therefore any operational incision contemplated in a person of this particular ethnic group should be carried out with the utmost care.

Ethnic Chinese. Port wine stains are said to be more common in this ethnic group. They are present at birth and are permanent − fortunately, most parents believe them to be a sign of good luck.

CULTURAL ISSUES

Cultural differences are a respectable entity and should not be mistaken for inequalities. If a cultural custom is thought to be the cause of a skin disease it should be discussed with the patient without any hint of denigration on the part of the doctor.

Arranged marriage and dowry. To preserve the extended family system, arranged marriages are an eastern custom. In Asian society a bridegroom is the breadwinner and is responsible for the maintenance of his wife and family. At the time of marriage, to help establish the newly-wedded couple, the bride's parents are obliged to make a financial contribution which is usually in the form of clothes, jewellery and household items − a dowry. In addition, all the wedding guests traditionally give cash and presents to the newlyweds, and at the same time examine the dowry which is on display.

Skin disease is considered a liability and has a direct influence on this system; this fact must be appreciated by a British GP. If a man has a skin disease it does not affect the dowry because he is expected to earn enough money for his own treatment, if it is private. However, it is not customary for the bride to earn her own living; therefore, if she has a skin disease, the bridegroom and his family have to pay for any required long-term treatment. As a result, the bride's parents feel morally obliged to give a larger dowry. A British doctor should reassure the parents that, under the NHS system, such treatment will be free and they will not have to face the expense of private treatment.

Medico-cultural problems. Cultural roots are very deep, and telling someone point-blank to stop a cultural habit will almost certainly fall on deaf ears: a compromise is therefore essential.

−   Some elderly Asians may have smallpox scars on their faces (Figure 3), something which a British doctor might never have seen before. Such patients have suffered an inferiority complex all their lives and any denigration, even inadvertently, will hurt their feelings.

−   Afro-Caribbean women and girls take pride in their intricately plaited hair which to them is a symbol of beauty. This may result in 'traction alopecia' due to excessive plaiting and should not be confused with 'alopecia areata' as the hair roots are still intact and the hair usually will grow again.

−   Most Asian women, especially those from Bangladesh, wear sandals, as shoes are considered masculine. It is not uncommon for such a patient to come to the surgery complaining of 'sandal chilblains'. They should be encouraged to wear warm socks in winter.

−   Nose-piercing is of cultural significance among Asians. A virgin girl may wear a nose-ring, whereas a married woman wears a nose-stud. Many barbers carry out nose-piercing in the UK. This form of self-adornment should not be frowned upon.

−   A British GP is used to seeing one or two boils on an English patient, but he may now be frequently confronted with an ethnic Asian or Afro-Caribbean patient, especially a child, who has just returned from a six-week summer holiday in his country of origin presenting with multiple boils ('heat boils') or their scars scattered all over the exposed areas of the body. These may mimic a mysterious tropical disease and are an extremely alarming sight to a teacher or a school nurse.

The temperatures in these tropical countries in mid-summer can often be as high as 120–130°F. Adults tend to stay indoors in such temperatures, but children often go outside to play, regardless of the intense heat. The dust and the profuse sweating makes the skin itchy, resulting in the inoculation of staphylococci by scratching. Other causative factors include minor injuries occurring in the presence of undernourishment, poor hygienic surroundings, and debilitating diseases such as malaria and dysentry. Some children will not eat the unusual local foods as they have been brought up on an English diet in Britain, and this leads to a lowered state of health.

Apart from the standard treatment for boils, all that is needed is positive reassurance to the parents and the school authorities that these boils are not leprotic or of a serious infectivity and that eventually the resulting scars will fade. Such a child should not be excluded from attending school, and the boils and scars should be kept covered so that other children are not frightened.

−   It is not uncommon for ethnic minority patients to visit the GP or the dermatologist and then go to an alternative therapist – a homoeopath, a *hakim*, a *vaid* or a faith healer (see Table 2 overleaf). Most alternative medical practitioners will ask the patient not to follow the GP's treatment at the same time, but the patient will not tell the GP that he is seeking alternative advice in case this annoys the GP. This occurrence is so common that I would suggest that a GP actively inquires about this and does not attempt to dissuade the patient, as such a patient will not comply. If a British doctor is understanding, the patient will feel free to return to him should any alternative remedy fail. A relevant case history will serve to illustrate the value of such advice.

A seven-year-old ethnic Indian boy was brought to the GP with an exacerbation of his eczema. The anxious parents demanded referral to a consultant dermatologist, expecting a fast, permanent cure. By the age of ten years the condition had not improved, so his parents consulted a homoeopath who instructed them to stop the GP's treatment and use homoeopathic remedies instead. As a result, a year later the condition had worsened and the boy's headteacher was so concerned that he referred the child to the school medical officer who decided to stop the homoeopathic treatment and send him to a special school by the coast. The parents were so annoyed at this that they sent him off to stay with his grandparents in India, where he received treatment from *hakims* and faith healers. At the age of 14 years, the boy returned to the UK, apparently cured, and returned to the same school after missing three valuable years of education. His recovery was consistent with the spontaneous resolution which can happen in this age group. It may or may not have been affected by any of the treatments. Better cultural understanding between the parents, the doctor, the dermatologist, the homoeopath, the headteacher and the school doctor could have saved all that wasted time, money and education.

Case histories such as this are common and illustrate that the importance of successful transcultural understanding cannot be overemphasised.

Table 2 *Alternative therapies popular among ethnic minorities*

Therapy	Medication	Therapeutic use
Hikmat – from a hakim (Muslim)	Herbal remedies (e.g. orally or locally) *Perhaiz* – hot or cold food	For many skin diseases (e.g. eczema) Avoidance of a certain food suspected causing allergy, for acute or chronic skin diseases (e.g. egg for eczema)
Folklore medicine – 'Granny's prescription'	Manual removal of head lice and nits by a relative	Pediculosis
	Sarsoon Ka Tail (sarsoon oil) locally	Dry skin (common in Asia due to prolonged sunshine)
	Coconut orally	Urticaria
	Poultice locally (with onions)	Boils
Holy medicine from a faith-healer (Hindu, Muslim, Catholic)	*Taveez* or *Mantra* – charms (holy words, written or read aloud)	Prevention and treatment of skin diseases
	Water (holy water from River Ganges or from Zamzam)	Psoriasis
	Warm air from mouth of a holy man after a short ritual	Chronic skin diseases and scorpion sting
Ayurvedic – from a *Vaid* (Hindu)	Elemental therapy	Chronic skin diseases
Homoeopathic – from a homoeopath, qualified or unqualified	Specific remedies	Eczema and other chronic skin diseases

NB. These therapies have an important bearing on the GP's medical treatment by interacting, potentiating or counteracting effects. Some alternative therapists forbid the concurrent use of the GP's treatment

SKIN PROBLEMS IN ASIANS:
AVOIDING THE DIAGNOSTIC TRAPS

The incidence and prevalence of certain skin conditions may show ethnic variations. In this section, the skin conditions peculiar to ethnic Asians – those living in the UK – are outlined and details of their cultural background which may be relevant to diagnosis and management are reviewed.

In her illuminating article (see note below on further reading), Dorothy Vollum demonstrated that dark skin may easily confuse the clinical picture in many dermatological problems. However, appearance is not the only problem here. Among ethnic Asians, some skin disorders seem to be more prevalent, and cultural differences, for example, diet or the use of cosmetics containing antimony or lead make the search for causes more wide-ranging.

Common skin disorders

There are a number of problems which appear to be more prevalent among ethnic Asian patients. An Asian male, for instance, may come to the surgery with a persistent eczematous lesion on one ankle. This condition is a form of neurodermatitis, and the standard treatment for eczema keeps it under control.

Tuberculosis of the skin and tubercular sinuses are common findings among ethnic Asians. The condition is a bovine tuberculosis to which Asians are said to be genetically predisposed. There may be no other symptoms of tuberculosis. A common site for such a sinus is the upper cervical region: it may be secondary to a solitary tuberculous lymph node.

Some children who go to India on holiday may return with scars from multiple body boils caused by the intensely hot weather. The scars last a long time but eventually disappear without need for any treatment. To those unfamiliar with the condition, they may indicate tropical diseases and result in patients being referred unnecessarily. Vitiligo is also common in ethnic Asians and may be a cause of distress.

At an immunisation session it may be noted that many ethnic Asian infants have a marked extensive blue discolouration on the buttock (Mongolian spots). This usually resolves within a few months without any treatment and should not be mistaken for bruises due to non-accidental injury.

Contact dermatitis may be seen in ethnic Asian women as a reaction to the surma (which has a lead content) used as a cosmetic of the tikka (containing antimony) applied as the red spot on the forehead.

Asians can be particularly prone to hirsuties, which can be a serious embarrassment for the adolescent girl. Her father may approach the GP because he is worried about its social consequences and his daughter's marriage prospects. The GP must understand the serious psychological effects of the condition and be prepared to recommend permanent removal of hair by electrolysis if shaving and waxing etc. prove unsatisfactory.

First published in *Modern Medicine*, **27**, No.3, March 1982, pp.28–29

Counselling

When diagnosing and prescribing for the ethnic Asian patient, it can be helpful to bear in mind his cultural background.

As many of the skin conditions are chronic, an ethnic Asian may be trying various other therapies in addition to the GP's orthodox medical treatment (see below). Some of these remedies may interact with, potentiate or counteract the drugs and lotions prescribed by the GP. The patient, however, will only tell the doctor if he asks and is seen to respect the patient's faith in alternative medicine.

As eczema may be related to a food allergy, the patient's diet needs to be considered. It may be relevant to know that many Gujaratis (West Indians) are vegetarians who eat eggs and milk, but some are vegans who do not. Vegans have loose motions which can affect the absorption of other food nutrients and some oral drugs.

The patient may believe that the GP does not understand him and that they are not on the same wavelength. This frustration at times manifests itself as direct aggression against the doctor or the receptionist.

On the other hand, an ethnic Asian will often tell his doctor what he thinks the doctor expects to hear, and this may be very different from the real circumstances of the case.

Popular folk remedies among ethnic Asians

- Herbal remedies (for many skin diseases eg, eczema) from the Hakim
- Perhaiz – avoidance of certain food suspected of causing allergy (for acute or chronic skin diseases, eg, eggs for eczema) from the Hakim
- Sarsoon oil locally (dry skin)
- Coconut oil locally (urticaria)
- Onion poultice locally (boils)
- Mantras or taveez – holy words, written or spoken, from a faith healer (prevention and treatment of skin diseases)
- Holy water from the Ganges (psoriasis)
- Warm breath from mouth of holy man after a short ritual (chronic skin diseases)
- Homoeopathy

ETHNIC CUSTOMS CAN AFFECT THE SKIN

Some Gujarati Hindus who come to the surgery, especially the elderly, may have religious tattoos around the neck, on the upper part of the chest and on the forearms.

A typical religious Hindu tattoo will look to the British GP like bunches of flowers mixed with clusters of swastikas. These tattoos represent the name of God (*Om*) in Hindi script which looks like a swastika, along with flowers, and other symbols, which are the names of relatives.

Some Europeans may have tattoos of statues and romantic messages almost anywhere on the body. Tattoos, as well as statues, are taboo in Islam, therefore a Muslim doctor may unwittingly take an instant dislike to such a patient. A female Asian doctor will shy away during an examination when she sees a tattooed message saying 'I love you'.

An understanding of the innocence of these tattoos is essential. An English trainer should not criticise an overseas graduate trainee for these reactions and should endeavour to aid understanding.

The snake is the symbol of knowledge in Europe, but it is a symbol of poisoning to most Asians. However, in some Asian cultures it is thought to be a symbol of God.

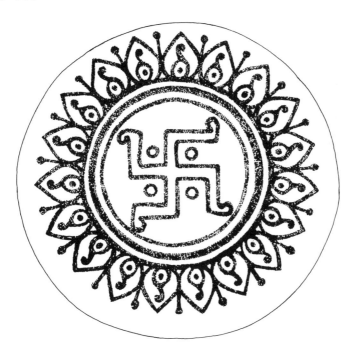

Swastika on a Hindu amulet

First published in *GP*, Sept. 28 1984, p.33 (Medical Publications Ltd.)

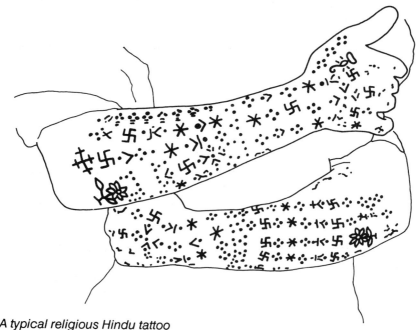

A typical religious Hindu tattoo

Prone to dark rings

Ethnic Asians are prone to dark rings around their eyes. It is not uncommon for an Asian mother to bring a female child to the GP for this reason because she may be worried that it will interfere with the girl's chances of a future arranged marriage.

She may be unaware of similar dark rings around her own eyes. The GP can reassure her that it obviously did not interfere with her own arranged marriage, and suggest a camouflage cream where necessary.

Shia Muslims live mainly in Iran, Iraq and Lebanon, and claim to be the descendants of the Prophet Mohammed. Every year they have a ceremony to mourn the anniversary of the murder of the Prophet's grandsons, Hasan and Hussain. Although all Muslims believe in the martyrdom of the innocent victims, it is only this section that carries out this ritual, which involves the beating of one's own chest and back with slaps and punches and even with sharp needles, chains and small knives. This annual ritual can result in bruising and scarring which will be reinforced each year. A person with such scars is considered holy by his peers. An English GP must never make adverse comments, and a casualty medical officer should not mistake these self-inflicted injuries for dermatitis artifacta, or other psychiatric conditions. In the case of an adolescent practising this ritual, the GP should explain the situation to a social worker who may otherwise mistake it for non-accidental injury.

An elderly Muslim male may develop callosity on his forehead due to excessive praying where the whole body weight is put on the forehead as it rests on the floor for prolonged periods. This is taken as a symbol of respect for his piousness by his family and no treatment is required.

Some Afro-Caribbeans also have ceremonial facial scars. These are more common in Africans than West Indians and in some tribes are considered to be a symbol of beauty.

A GP may see some ethnic minority patients with a contact dermatitis caused by allergy to metals, including silver and gold. Ethnic dress such as saris and kurtas may be made of material threaded with silver or gold. Tikka (a red spot on the forehead) worn by Hindu women, and sandoor, worn along the hair parting by married Hindu women, are made of antimony. Surma contains lead and is customarily applied to the eyelids of Asian children and women, especially for religious festivals. Rakhi is an armband tied ceremoniously by a Hindu sister on her brother's arm on 'Brother's Day', and is sometimes made of metal.

Muslims, especially Malaysians, are very fond of wearing charms, some holy words written on paper sealed in a tiny metal box that is worn on a chain around the neck or arm. A GP, after diagnosing, should discuss with them a substitute which can be worn instead of that particular metal.

Ethnic Afro-Caribbeans, especially children, are more likely to develop traction alopecia due to excessive plaiting. Elderly English women may develop this condition because of sleeping in hair curlers.

Some English women (and men) dye their hair in various colours and some adolescents may have multicoloured hair. This may appear strange to a newcomer to western society.

To disguise grey hair, an Asian woman will dye her hair (and an Asian man, his beard) red, using henna. This may appear strange to an English GP. Many Asian girls, especially brides, dye their palms, soles and nails with henna (Mehndi), making flower patterns.

It is said that if one parent is blond and the other dark-haired, their child will be a redhead. If an English blond girl marries a dark-haired Cypriot who may be unaware of this possibility, the birth of a red-headed baby may arouse his suspicions of her infidelity. Morbid jealousy is more common in ethnic Greeks, Turks, Cypriots and Italians. In such a case a GP can help this family by positive reassurance.

If a red-headed mother with a lot of freckles marries a dark-haired man, it is possible that the child may have individual clusters of freckles which may mimic a skin disease. A GP running an infant welfare clinic should bear this in mind.

In chronic conditions it is not uncommon for an ethnic minority patient to turn to alternative medicine. Some parents who do not comply with GP/specialist treatment for their child's eczema turn to complementary medicine and fail. Such a situation can be avoided by a better rapport between the doctor and the patient.

Poverty, ignorance and disease are norms of the third world. Because these problems are insoluble in their cultures, eastern patients (and doctors) may have no concept of the social aspects of a problem. They consider social problems none of the GP's business. No GP could practise good medicine in a transcultural setting without bridging this gap.

SKIN PROBLEMS IN MULTI-ETHNIC GROUPS

The colour of normal skin originates from melanin, oxyhaemoglobin, reduced haemoglobin, and carotene. Melanin results from an enzymatic oxidation of tyrosine by tyrosinase, which is attached to the melanocytes at the epidermo-dermal junction. See below.

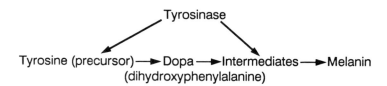

Melamin pigment is produced by neural crest cells (melanocytes) which normally migrate to the levels of the germinal layer of the epidermis. There they manufacture melanin pigment granules which are injected into the epidermal cells by means of fine dendritic processes.

Ethnic pigmentation of the skin is determined by the quality of melanin, produced by melanocytes which are present in equal numbers in all races. An excessive quantity of melanin pigment may have pathological significance. For example, in dark skin even mild inflammation causes excessive pigment formation which may be very slow to fade.

The factors influencing melanin production are:

Internal	External
Melanocyte-stimulating hormone (MSH) (anterior pituitary) in alpha and beta forms	Sun
	Stress
Steroids (adrenal cortex)	
Melanocytes (skin)	

The role of MSH in man is unknown, but I would suggest it could be related to melanin regulation. However, at present steroids are accepted to be responsible for this.

The chief function of melanisation is the prevention of ultra-violet photolysis of folate and other light-sensitive nutrients. Recent studies suggest that *in vitro* human plasma loses 30–50% of folate in 60 minutes in strong sunlight. *In vivo*, patients treated with ultra-violet light show abnormally low folate levels. Consequently it is reasonable to believe that, given the same level of exposure to the sun in the UK, various ethnic groups will present with different patterns of skin disease.

This material first published in *1983 RCGP Members' Reference Book*, 1983, pp.389–393 (Royal College of General Practitioners)

Some clinical problems in general practice

In general practice, patients sometimes present with specific skin problems which become diagnostic traps for the unwary.

Ethnic English. Acne cosmetica on the face may be induced by repeated application of creams by fashion-conscious English women. There is compelling evidence that sunlight produces skin cancer, especially basal and squamous cell carcinoma, in people who have less melanin pigment. Melanomas are also related to sun exposure but in a more complicated way. Lesions on exposed areas of skin in ethnic English patients who have been abroad in hot climates for any length of time should, therefore, be regarded with suspicion, and a diagnosis should not be delayed.

Ethnic Asians. Some skin disorders seem to be more prevalent among ethnic Asians. Cultural differences – for example, diet, or the use of cosmetics containing antimony or lead – make the search for causes more difficult. For example, an Asian male may come to the surgery with a persistent eczamatous lesion on one ankle. This condition is a form of neurodermatitis and needs the appropriate treatment.

Tuberculosis of the skin and tubercular sinuses are common findings among ethnic Asians. The condition is a bovine tuberculosis to which Asians are said to be genetically predisposed. Another reason could be a brief holiday visit of an Asian to India where he drinks fresh cow's milk. The cow, being sacred in India, escapes the rigorous control of anti-tubercular vaccination in some areas, and cow's milk in Asia is not usually pasteurised. There may be no other symptons of tuberculosis. A common site for such a sinus is the upper cervical region; it may be secondary to a solitary tuberculous lymph node.

Vitiligo is also common in ethnic Asians and may be a cause of considerable distress, especially when the traditional arranged marriage is affected.

Ethnic Asian women who become pregnant or use oral contraceptives are more likely to get cloasma – a dark brown discolouration on both sides of the face, below the eyelids. Cosmetic cream may conceal it, but these women may ask for a cure from the general practitioners because the lesion persists, even after they have stopped taking oral contraceptives, and in such cases supportive counselling will be required.

Ethnic Afro-Caribbeans. Sparseness of hair in some black children may be mistaken for alopecia areata. However, in an adolescent girl, alopecia areata may be induced due to excessive plaiting of the hair.

Ceremonial scars on the face of an African woman may be noted while no such scars are present in ethnic West Indian women, and one may inadvertently hurt the woman's feelings by criticising the scars. Keloid scars after burns are more common in Afro-Caribbean patients, who have a racial pre-disposition to these.

It is interesting to note that head lice change colour according to the colour of the patient's scalp. Thus head lice in Afro-Caribbean patients are black, whereas in Asian patients they are brown, and in English patients, pink.

Industrial dermatitis is reported to be less common in Afro-Caribbeans (and Asians). On the other hand, acne cosmetica, due to pomades and creams, induces acneiform changes particularly in Afro-Caribbeans.

Ethnic Chinese. Port wine stains are apparently more common among the Chinese population. It has also been reported that fungal infections between the fingers and toes occur more among Chinese adults, perhaps because many Chinese work in the hot and moist atmosphere of the kitchen in their family-run restaurants.

Ethnic Cypriots. Greek or Turkish – or African – patients may report with leg ulcers which may be due to sickle cell disease. They should be investigated and the appropriate treatment instituted. These lesions should not be mistaken for varicose or eczematous ulcers.

Multitherapy

Many ethnic minority patients may be using other therapies in addition to the treatment prescribed by the general practitioner. For example, a Chinese patient may go to an acupuncturist. A West Indian may be using coconut oil locally for urticaria or a poultice locally for boils, and various spiritualist treatments. Especially in view of the recent increase in prescription charges, many ethnic English patients will try over-the-counter remedies. Such multitherapy may result in partial or complete non-compliance on the part of the patient, and interaction or counter-action of a drug, prescribed by the doctor.

General practitioner consultations

When diagnosing and prescribing for multi-ethnic patients, the doctor may find it helpful to bear in mind their cultural backgrounds. As many skin conditions are chronic, an ethnic minority patient may be trying various other therapies in addition to the general practitioner's treatment. Some of these remedies may interact, potentiate, or counteract the orthodox drugs and lotions prescribed. The patient, however, will only tell the doctor if he asks, and if he is seen to respect the patient's faith in alternative medicine.

As eczema may be related to a food allergy, the patient's diet needs to be considered. Moreover, vegans have loose motions which can affect the absorption of other food nutrients and some oral drugs. The consequences of various diets and dietary habits must be borne in mind.

Obviously, when a doctor is dealing with multi-ethnic patients, he needs more patience and tact than when he is counselling patients of a single culture. Patience is a virtue in general practice, especially in the management of chronic skin problems.

A multi-ethnic approach to the diagnosis and management of skin problems should be at the forefront of current medical thinking. Failure to take this into consideration may lead to diagnostic pitfalls and unnecessary morbidity.

Further reading

Cohen, A. (1981). Sun, sea and skin cancer. *Doctor*, 4 June, 24

Cotterill, J.A. (1982). Acne. *Practitioner*, **226**, 1227–1236

du Vivier, A. (1982). Skin cancer – new cure for early changes. *General Practitioner*, 22 October, 55

Hawk, J. (1982). Skin cancer/prevention. *General Practitioner*, 22 October, 51

Hawk, J. (1982). The effects of sunlight on the skin. *Practitioner*, **226**, 1258–1266

Levene, G.M. and Calnan, C.D. (1974). *A Colour Atlas of Dermatology*. Wolfe Medical Books

Monk, B. (1983). How to spot a malignant melanoma. *Pulse*, 5 February, 57

Smith, T.C.G. (1982). General Practice comment – dermatology. *Practitioner*, **226**, 1350

Solomons, B. (1973). *Lecture Notes on Dermatology*, 3rd Edn. London, Blackwell Scientific Publications

Vollum, D.I. (1981). An illustrated guide to dermatoses in dark skin. *Modern Medicine*, November, 32–37

Woodward, J. (1981). A 'healthy' tan holds hidden dangers. *Pulse*, 20 June, 53

Part III
SELECTED POINTS

CHAPTER 26

MULTI-CULTURAL MEDICINE: A SERIES IN THE BRITISH MEDICAL JOURNAL

Hooka – The hooka is a smoking apparatus: a flask half filled with water is connected through a pipe to an earthenware funnel containing tobacco paste, which is covered with a stone disc over which there are lighted coals; another pipe from the side of the flask above the water level is connected to a mouthpiece. As with the chestpiece of a stethoscope, this mouthpiece is never sterilised. One person inhales the smoke that originates from the tobacco paste filtered through the water through the mouthpiece, and then it is passed to the next person and so on among the family, relatives, and visitors, who sit around in a circle most evenings after dinner for a 'pow-wow'. This custom is popular not only in the Asian subcontinent but also with Arabs, Iranians, Chinese, and south east Asians. This was a sight familiar to British Army personnel when visiting these areas. This form of smoking is as dangerous as any other and its use should be elicited through direct questioning. The Sikh religion, however, forbids smoking, and to a devout Sikh this would be an offensive question. Therefore an indirect approach is more tactful.

Betel (pan) chewing – This is a unique Asian habit – an after dinner delicacy – enjoyed by a tenth of the world's population. Its ingredients have a great psychological value. After all, cultural habits are based on the so called scientific thinking of when they originated. The betel leaf is a source of vitamin C. The betel nut is an astringent. Limestone paste (calcium hydroxide) is a rich source of calcium and stimulates salivation. Catechu is not only an astringent but also a source of iron. Rose hips contain vitamin C and have a pleasant taste. Tumeric is used for colouring and silver foil is thought to be aphrodisiac. Every betel seller will ask the customer whether he would like betel with or without tobacco. Most will choose tobacco. A few may choose to try additional 'special ingredients', which may be hard drugs such as cocaine, LSD (lysergide), etc.

The results of recent studies have shown that oral cancers are more common in ethnic minority groups, and carcinoma of the cheek is most common among the betel chewing population[1,2]. betel chewing may be responsible for this in two ways. Firstly, an unspecified amount of tobacco is kept against the inside of the cheek for long periods. This may affect the buccal mucosa directly. Secondly,

First published in *British Medical Journal*, **290**, 1985, pp.1632, 1956; **291**, 1985, pp.790, 872, 1020; **294**, 1985, p.160; **295**, 1985, pp.818,890 limestone paste (calcium hydroxide), if not mixed sufficiently with water, has an abrasive action and can cause an ulcer which may become chronic and develop carcinogenic changes, resulting in cancer of the cheek.

Ackee – This fruit is a delicacy in Jamaica and is used in 'bush tea', The ripe fruit can be eaten after a meal without ill effects, but if it is unripe it may be poisonous. It may cause hypoglycaemia due to two factors: hypoglycin A and hypoglycin B. This may result in vomiting (Jamaican vomiting sickness), coma, and even death due to severe dehydration. Three quarters of the West Indians who live in the United Kingdom have come from Jamaica. They often go home on holiday and bring tinned ackee back with them, which may contain unripe fruit.

Ginger bezoars – Preserved ginger root is a popular Chinese snack and, if it is not chewed properly or is eaten in a hurry, can cause small bowel obstruction at the ileocaecal junction. The ginger root consists of cellulose, which is resistant to gastric juices, absorbs water, and swells up during transit through the gut. An elderly Chinese adult patient or a child may complain of pain in the right iliac fossa. This must be considered in the differential diagnoses of acute abdomen.

Teeth grinding – The British believe that this is a psychological symptom but Iranians believe otherwise. They think that grinding the teeth is a symptom of threadworm infestation. An ethnic Iranian father may bring his child to a British doctor with this problem, expecting to get a stool examination to diagnose helminthiasis, and will be disappointed if this is not done. Mutual understanding is required.

Mongolian spots and culture – This is an ethnic characteristic. These congenital, macular, and non-inflammatory patches are common in ethnic Asian infants – Indian, Pakistani, Bangladeshi, and Sri Lankan. These are not uncommon in Afro-Caribbeans, especially West Indians (in the West Indies there is 'an African as well as Asian' population). Occasionally these are noted in Eskimos and Europeans of Celtic origin, especially those with dark hair. They are collections of spindle shaped melanocytes located deep in the dermis. These are blue, slate grey, or black, commonly occuring in the sacral region but may occur anywhere on the skin, including the face. These spots vary in shape and size. Some can resemble finger marks and mimic a bruise. The colour usually fades during the first year and they disappear by the end of the first decade. No treatment is required. The cause is unknown, thus more research is needed. It is important not to confuse them with bruises as the condition is often mistaken for a bruise if it has not been seen before. Many British general practitioners, health visitors, and consultant paediatricians in the National Health Service, especially those from South Africa, may never have examined an Asian or Afro-Caribbean infant.

In Asian culture to secure the extended family system, marriages are arranged – the less you see of the others, the more you stick to one – and the husband is often more loyal to his mother than to his wife. A woman is expected to give birth to a spotless baby, especially if it is a male. It is not surprising, therefore, that the mother may feel guilty and believe that this Mongolian spot is her genetic failure. The mother-in-law, who believed when she was young that her own mother-in-law was awful and now thinks that her daughter-in-law is horrible, might think of it as a curse and be ready to blame the mother. A general practitioner should not only reassure the mother, but also explain this to the family.

Fuel can be added to the fire when an English health visitor sees such an infant on her first visit and suspects child abuse. The mother-in-law may collude with her and, despite the mother's denials and tears, she calls a 'case conference' to be chaired by a consultant paediatrician. The general practitioner, unlike the consultant, is not salaried and is paid on a 'service per item' basis, and, knowing that there is no fee for such an attendance, carries on looking after his sick patients, and declines the invitation to attend, and no wonder. A lot of time and money is wasted.

If every medical student, general practitioner trainee, and health visitor could be shown such cases, much expense, stress and tears could be avoided.

Eye-to-eye contact – There is more to it than meets the eye. In Western culture looking someone in the eye is a good thing and during a conversation constant eye to eye contact is desirable. Lack of eye-to-eye contact while talking is considered rude as it is supposed to show shiftiness and an indication to break contact. The Germans will have such piercing eye-to-eye contact that even the English will shy away.

The reverse is the case in Eastern culture. To look someone in the eye is rude and after an initial and intermittent eye to eye contact, to look away during a conversation is, in fact, a sign of respect. An ethnic Asian, Chinese, and Afro-Caribbean – whether a doctor or a patient – will look away when talking to an English doctor or patient as a sign of respect. An English patient should not be annoyed if an Asian doctor looks away while listening, and an English doctor should never keep looking in the eye of an Afro-Caribbean or Chinese woman, especially in front of her husband. An English man should not make eyes at an Indian woman doctor, especially in her surgery! It could be very embarrassing.

Thumbs up – Clear non-verbal communication between a doctor and his patient is essential for good rapport. If a consultant or a general practitioner of one ethnic group communicates with a patient of another it is essential to know that they have correctly interpreted the sign language. Thumbs up symbolises 'OK' or success in Britain and North America, but it is considered a very rude sign by Belgians, Greeks, and Asians, and is equal to swearing. Just imagine what could happen when a Greek Cypriot or an Indian patient consults an English doctor. At the end of a very successful consultation, the doctor gives him the thumbs up sign!

Spitting and culture – A practice, if everyone is doing it – even if it is wrong – becomes socially acceptable. In the West, smoking has been very popular and the general practitioner either provided an ash tray or put a notice 'No Smoking Please' in their waiting rooms. In the Asian subcontinent and Greece, however, spitting on the ground is a social habit. In Eastern culture 'betel chewing' is popular and it is customary in general practice surgeries to provide a 'peek-dan' (a receiver) or a health education talk.

The World Health Organisation has been organising 'anti-spitting' weeks in the third world countries. Spitting is detested in Europe, but the ingestion of saliva is considered nauseating in Asia and Africa. There is a conflict where these two cultures meet which, I believe, may be avoided by mutual understanding. In Bradford, where many ethnic Pakistanis live, there are notices in Asian languages in public places 'Spitting is forbidden'. The London Borough of Ealing is tough and in Southall, where there is a large population of ethnic Indians, the notices on lamp posts read in English only 'Spitting on Footways: Penalty £50'.

In Britain, a private practitioner will probably opt for providing a 'peek-dan' or receiver but an NHS general practitioner may choose to put a notice 'No Spitting Please'. Nevertheless, the importance of health education cannot be over emphasised.

Indian six-week rule – A British general practitioner was surprised when a young Indian mother with her first-born child after his check up at six weeks said, 'I am so pleased, doctor because today he is 6 weeks old, and I can now dress him in new clothes'. When the doctor asked her, 'Why not before now?' she told him that according to centuries-old Indian tradition a mother is not supposed to buy her baby new clothes for six weeks after birth and that she has to borrow old clothes from relatives and friends. She could not give any reason for this and did not know anyone else who could. I suggest that this could be because neonatal deaths were so common in Indian villages that new clothes were considered not to be worth buying until the baby's hold on life was firmly established.

Another Indian tradition should also be remembered. A new mother is not supposed to take her baby out for 40 days, possibly to avoid the risk of infection from outside contacts. During this period relatives and friends visit the mother but often are not given the chance to see the new baby. After 40 days, however, the mother is expected to visit all her relatives, taking the baby with her in its new clothes, and she may be too shy to breast feed it outside her new home.

An English health visitor or doctor visiting the new baby may inadvertently interpret these points as signs of child neglect or even child abuse. Such a health worker should not hesitate to ask the mother tactfully for an explanation and should not insist on her bringing the baby to the clinic before six weeks are up as long as the mother and baby are found to be well at home visits.

Animal oil – A high caste Hindu mother complained to her Irish general practitioner at her baby's six week check up, that she was very upset because she gave milk A on the advice of the English ward sister in the maternity hospital. But she subsequently learnt from her Muslim health visitor that it contained beef extract, which is taboo in the Hindu religion. She changed to milk B, which is for vegetarians, but was angry and guilty of polluting her baby's religion. She vowed never to attend that maternity hospital again. The general practitioner was sympathetic and reassuring, and he spoke to the health visitor, pleading with her to soften her advice. The health visitor told him that she could not hide the truth as it was Ramadan, and she showed him the containers of milk A which contained 'animal oil' and milk B which did not. Respecting her feelings the general practitioner wrote to the manufacturers, who said that animal oil is in fact cow's fat, which is added to skimmed milk to make it more like breast milk. The doctor came across a Muslim mother who read the contents which included animal oil. She was convinced that it could only be pork extract, which is taboo in the Muslim religion, and she had therefore used milk B. The Catholic midwife told her not to trust anyone and just breast feed, but she was unable to breast feed.

A doctor should never recommend a milk containing animal oil – which is beef fat – to a Hindu mother and should not hide the truth because the mother has to live with the terrible guilt feeling and cultural misunderstanding when she finds out. Patients are better informed than we may think.

Tale of the unexpected – An English doctor in Harley Street told his Polish secretary not to dry her hands with the towel in the examination room. She looked suspiciously at the doctor, wondering what on earth had gone on the previous evening after she had left him examining an affluent Arab traveller. The doctor explained that the towel had been used by the patient as 'shorts'. He said that after taking the history and checking the patient's bare chest, he had asked the chap to slip his trousers down and pop up on the couch for examination of the abdomen. When he looked up after making notes he was horrified to see the bearded man standing stark naked with his genitalia shrivelled up with embarrassment. The doctor was taken aback but gave him the surgery towel. 'He looked civilised and was wearing a Western suit; but how terrible, he wasn't wearing underpants'. Muttering these words, the doctor left. And the secretary wondered 'Why on earth...'.

In Eastern cultures, especially in the tropics, it is customary not to wear underpants and for both men and women to shave pubic hair. This ensures personal hygiene by avoiding the sweat which can act as a sort of superglue. Only Sikhs wear underpants and have uncut hair, which is part of their faith, and they keep it scrupulously clean. Of course, an Eastern doctor will be equally surprised when examining a Western patient. Indeed, though Westernised, a doctor from the East may retain some Eastern habits and concepts.

'A state of nakedness in modern Western society is extremely unusual. Since it is likely that more patients will be undressing more often in general practice, the subject of nakedness in medicine seems worthy of careful analysis and understanding.'(Denis Pereira-Gray) In Eastern society a person rarely undresses in front of a spouse, let alone a stranger. Many cross-cultural innocent misunderstandings may be avoided by preparing oneself for such a transcultural encounter – the occupational hazard of modern health professionals.

References

1. Burton-Bradley, B.G. (1979). Is betel-chewing carcinogenic? *Lancet*, ii, 903
2. Anonymous. (1985). Views. *Br. Med. J.*, 290, 940

CHAPTER 27

TRANSCULTURAL MEDICINE: EDUCATION AND EXAMINATION

PATIENT CARE, CRICKET AND TRANSCULTURAL CONFUSION

What possible connection has the almost 'international incident' between Mike Gatting, captain of the England cricket team, and Shakoor Rana, the Pakistani umpire, got to do with what goes on in a GP's surgery?

The incident was a classic example of how the light at the end of the tunnel for a person from one culture is the headlamp of an oncoming train for someone from another.

Shakoor Rana, seeing that Mike Gatting was moving a fielder as the bowler started his run-up, waved his index finger in a vertical plane, looked Gatting in the eye and in a loud voice announced: 'Hold on, that's cheating.' Gatting retorted: 'You bloody cheat, keep your mouth shut', and showed the well-known two-fingers-up sign.

Gatting was later told to give an unconditional written apology. To show his contempt, while obeying orders, he handed over the apology written on a tatty piece of paper.

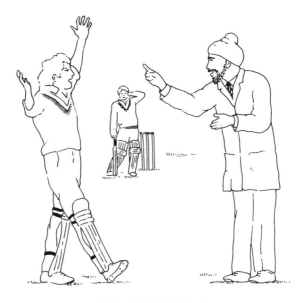

First published in *Pulse*, **48**, No.31, July 30 1988, p.36 (Morgan Grampian Professional Press)

If the umpire had been Dicky Bird, the venue Lords and not Faisalabad, the scene would have been different. The umpire would have wagged his finger from side to side and said: 'Hold on – that's not quite right.'

There is no equivalent in the Pakistani language for 'fair play' and so the word 'cheating' is quite acceptable. In Eastern cultures, using the index finger is normal during conversation. But by looking someone in the eye and speaking loudly, gestures which are acceptable in Western culture, Shakoor Rana would have been seen as rude by Pakistanis.

Gatting's reply was offensive because he did not respect the umpire's authority. Also the word 'bloody', while common among Westerners, is a great insult to a Pakistani. The two-finger sign was neither here nor there as it is considered amusing if done by a European.

In Eastern culture any form of written apology is preferable to a verbal one and is kept as a souvenir. Writing on a tatty piece of paper is not an insult, the recipient merely feels sorry for the sender who presumably was very poor!

What parochial lesson can be learnt from this international debacle? Consider these next case histories – all examples where offence unwittingly was given and dysfunctional consultations ensued.

Health visitor's thumbs-up

An English health visitor brought a Punjabi woman (non-English speaking) to see a south Indian woman doctor in a family planning clinic. They were assisted by a Kenyan-Asian interpreter.

Just before leaving, the health visitor showed a thumbs-up sign to reassure the patient that she was in good hands. The Punjabi woman blushed and covered her face with both hands in embarrassment.

The interpreter explained that 'thumb-up', especially with a lateral or vertical movement, is a very rude sign in Asian culture.

The winking professor

A 30-year-old Bangladeshi woman who was suffering with migraine was taken by her husband to see an English neurologist at a teaching hospital. During history-taking and examination, the doctor kept winking to the woman to reassure here, as she spoke only Bengali.

The patient and her husband left the consulting room in disgust, without waiting for any investigations or advice and complained to their GP.

In the East, winking at a woman is an invitation to go to bed.

The misunderstood speech therapist

A young Sikh boy was referred to an Australian speech therapist by a Cockney schoolteacher with the complaint that he would not speak to her.

The therapist found his speech normal but perceived a hearing defect because in answering some questions, he said 'I don't hear you, Miss!'

The GP – who was familiar with such complaints – examined his hearing and found it to be normal.

The mystery was solved when the GP went to the school and, speaking to the teacher, explained that an Asian child – unless very Westernised – would not communicate when embarrassed.

If compelled to answer a question by a teacher or health professional that he did not understand, a child would say politely, 'I did not hear', because to say 'I did not understand you' is very rude in Asian culture.

BOOK REVIEW

As she is spoke

English in Medicine. A Course in Communication Skills. E. H. Glendenning, B. A. S. Holstrom. (160 pp; figs; coursebook £4.75 paperback, plus complementary cassette £8.62 inc. VAT.) Cambridge: Cambridge University Press, 1987. ISBN coursebook 0-521-31165-9, cassette 0-521-32332-0.

Good communication skills are essential for establishing a better doctor – patient rapport. The last thing a patient – the most important person in medicine – needs is a doctor who cannot communicate, even if he or she is a medical wizard. The criterion of good English, according to Bill Whimster, is that it 'should be spoken or written in such a way that it sounds infallibly English to English ears'. This English language course also covers English customs and medical etiquette necessary in caring for British patients, especially those from south-east England.

Written by Cambridge teachers with vast experience in teaching English to medical professionals in Britain, this intermediate level course adopts a student-centered approach – suitable both for classroom use and private study – and covers written and recorded interviews dealing with history taking, examination, investigations, diagnosis, explanation, and treatment. The text is easily readable, full of factual information, includes clear illustrations based on actual case notes, and contains some authentic articles of practical use for the PLAB test.

The cassette demonstrates a true English accent. English is, of course, spoken with many accents throughout the world. Some doctors from Scotland, Wales, Cornwall, Devonshire, Yorkshire, and the north speak with such broad accents that they find it difficult to understand each other. Moreover, accent and colloquial content vary between all English-speaking countries, even between the United Kingdom and the United States. 'The English have really everything in common with the Americans except, of course, the language' (Oscar Wilde). For example, Durex is called a condom in Britain and a rubber in the USA – and it is named as Sellotape in Australia: mind your language when visiting a stationery shop. Nevertheless. a reader should learn to understand the English accent without losing his own, and to make himself understood.

First published in *British Medical Journal,* **294**, 1987, p.1607

The book is written for all those who learn English as a second language and wish to care for English patients. There could, however, be some interesting misunderstandings if a doctor were to go by this book when dealing with patients from other cultures. The question 'Do you drink?' implies alcohol to British patients, but it means soft drinks to an Asian, (Hindu, Sikh, or Muslim) or a Chinese (Buddhist) patient. Another question, 'And any problems with your waterworks?' will make an English patient describe his urinary complaints, but an oriental patient may start talking about that dreadful freezing and subsequent bursting of the pipes in the house last winter. Finally, when a doctor says, 'Would you slip off your top things, please?' it makes sense to an English patient but an Asian woman won't have a clue. She will keep nodding her head – a sign which to an English doctor denotes understanding – and it may be some time before both realise that they misunderstood each other.

In addition to colloquial English the course highlights three things: first, an English patient often uses cliches such as 'Well, doctor,' 'You see', 'You know', and takes his time when describing his or her illness. Second, an English doctor explains everything that he does to a patient. Finally, when giving a prognosis, an English doctor remains non-committal and in making decisions he includes not only the patient but also the relatives.

Britain receives many doctors – a legacy of the British empire – from the Commonwealth. Many British medical bodies like examining their skills but hardly anyone wants to educate them adequately. 'It is one thing to show a man he is in error, it is another to put him in possession of truth' (John Locke). This course is therefore an essential purchase for new overseas graduates, despite their financial difficulties, and because of its wider appeal it should be kept in all medical libraries, at home and abroad.

MODERN MEDICINE POSTGRADUATE PROMPTCARD

The Royal College of General Practitioners approves of the use of Promptcards for vocational training and continuing medical education.

Transcultural medicine comprises the medical encounters between a doctor or health worker of one ethnic group and a patient of another. It embraces the physical, psychological and social aspects of care, communication, as well as religious, ethnic and cultural issues.

1. Which foods and drinks are forbidden for those with a variety of religious convictions and what practical problems might these present for the general practitioner? For example, alcohol is taboo for muslims and many proprietary medicines contain alcohol.

2. Avoidance of eye-to-eye contact is a sign of respect in eastern cultures. What practical problems may arise in connection with this when a Chinese woman consults you? How would you overcome this?

3. Discuss how the higher incidence of umbilical hernias and hydroceles in certain ethnic groups might affect paediatric surveillance in general practice.

4. Acetylator status varies according to ethnic origin. There are more slow acetylators in ethnic minority groups. Consider how this could influence your prescribing habits. For which groups of drugs is this knowledge important?

5. Mongolian spots are more common in Asians. An English health visitor suspects non-accidental injury and calls a case conference. Discuss the implications of her action.

6. Discuss how much you should learn about the ethnic minorities represented in your practice and how you will do this.

Further reading

Freedman (1984). Caucasian (letter). *Br. Med. J.*, 696
Pietroni (1976). Non-verbal communication in GP surgery. Chapter 10 in: Tanner (ed.) *Language and Communication in General Practice*. Hodder and Stoughton

First published as *Modern Medicine Promptcard*, Sept. 1984

APPENDIX 1

RESOURCES AVAILABLE

LOCAL

- Priest / Rabbi / Imam / Pandit / Guru
- Racial Equality Council
- Interpreter / Linkperson / Relative / Friend
- MP / Councillor / Community Worker / Leader

NATIONAL

- Commission for Racial Equality
- Appropriate embassy / DOH
- Voluntary organisations
- Cultural, religious or ethnic helplines

Note: Any doctor or health professional may seek advice from any of the above sources and it is expected that the advice will be free on any cultural, religious and ethnic issue.

DISPOSAL OF THE DEAD AND MOURNING CUSTOMS

Table 1 Customs for disposal of the dead

Religion/persuasion	Burial	Cremation	Who can touch the body?
Anglicans	Acceptable	Acceptable	Any health professional/authorized person
Catholics	Preferred	No prohibition	ditto
Jehovah's Witnesses	Acceptable	Acceptable	ditto
Mormons	Preferred	Frowned upon	ditto
Christian Scientists	No prohibition	Preferred	Persons of same sex. Others should wear gloves
Africans/Caribbeans	Acceptable	Acceptable	Any health professional. A black sister preferred
Rastafarians	Preferred	No prohibition	ditto
Jews	Preferred by Orthodox	Preferred by Liberals	Specially trained Jews or family members of the same sex. Others should wear gloves
Muslims	Always	Never	Family members of the same sex. Others should wear gloves
Hindus	Never	Always	ditto
Sikhs	Infants only	All adults	ditto
Buddhists	Rare	Usual	Any health professional/authorized person
Baha'is	Always	Never	ditto
Zoroastrians (Parsees)	Neither (left in Tower of Silence in India)	Neither (one cemetery in Britain)	ditto
Atheists/Agnostics	Acceptable	Preferred	ditto

Table 2 *Mourning customs*

Mourners' religion or persuasion	Minimum period of mourning	Mourners' dress colour	Hair cut shaving	Public expression of grief
Christians	Unspecified	Black	Not applicable	Low key/stoic
Jews	7 days	Black	Beards not shaved for 7 days	Lamenting essential. Professional mourners invited
Muslims	3 days (widow for 130 days)	Black (but in Iran the paler brown)	Not applicable	Low key to lamenting, and reading the Holy Quran
Hindus	10 – 13 days	White	No hair cut for males and widow's head shaved on 3rd day	Lamenting and chanting from sacred scriptures
Sikhs	10 days	White	Hair is normally uncut	Low key, and reading from the Holy Guru Granth
Buddhists	Unspecified	White (especially Chinese)	Widow's head shaved on 3rd day in Japan	Lamenting and all night vigil. Chanting prayers. Professional mourners invited
Atheists	Unspecified	Black	Not applicable	Low key/stoic or party to celebrate life of deceased
Royals	Unspecified	Purple/violet	Not applicable	Low key/stoic
Black Christian Americans	Unspecified	Yellow	Not applicable	Low key to lamenting
Black Africans	8 days (widows 1 year)	Black	Widow's head shaved. Widower's head shaved and beard grown (8 days)	Loud wailing cry collectively

EXAMINATION QUESTIONS

(For Essays or MEQs)

Q1. Russian Orthodox Jewish parents take their child, who suffers from Tay – Sachs disease, to see an English male doctor in Oxford. Culture, religion and ethnicity are important environmental and genetic factors. What transcultural encounters are likely to occur in history-taking, examination, diagnosis, management and compliance?

Q2. A Somali (African) Muslim woman, suffering from anxiety – depression, consults a Scottish male doctor in Glasgow. Culture, religion and ethnicity affect the presentation and management of a disease. What transcultural encounters are likely to occur in history-taking, examination, diagnosis, management and compliance?

Q3. An Oxbridge Englishman, presented with symptoms of pernicious anaemia and enlarged prostate, consults an Asian Hindu, overseas qualified, woman doctor in London. Culture, religion and ethnicity have important influence on medical consultation. What transcultural encounters might occur in history-taking, examination, diagnosis, management and compliance?

Q4. A Greek Cypriot man consults with a tweedy English lady doctor. He wonders whether his wife-to-be (not present at the consultation) can be checked out as her brother had a funny blood disease which deformed him and led to his death in childhood. He wants his children to be strong.

Q5. A middle-aged red-headed Irishman from County Clare is brought to the doctor by his sister because of a cut on his head. He smells of alcohol. There is a past history of admission to a psychiatric hospital. His sister says he is getting more strange and she cannot put up with his drinking. The doctor is an Iraqi exile. How might culture affect the consultation?

Q6. A Nigerian woman presents her two-year-old son to her Ulster-born GP with a swollen wrist. The child was crying and in a lot of pain. There were two older children with the lady. She denied that her son had fallen. What cultural aspects might affect this consultation?

Multiple Choice Questions

1. Transcultural Medicine is concerned with:

A.   ethnic minorities
B.   different cultures
C.   anthropological issues
D.   medical problems
E.   biological differences

2. In an African the colour of the retina is:

A.   pink
B.   black
C.   chocolate brown
D.   blue
E.   red

3. This concerns oral contraceptive pill-induced hypertension. Rank the following ethnic groups in the frequency of this condition:

A.   Europeans
B.   Asians
C.   Caribbeans
D.   Africans
E.   Chinese

4. Pork insulin is acceptable to:

A.   Christians
B.   Orthodox Jews
C.   Devout Muslims
D.   Hindus
E.   Sikhs

5. Antibiotics in capsules (gelatine) are acceptable to:

A. Vegetarians
B. Orthodox Jews
C. Liberal Muslims
D. Devout Hindus
E. Buddhists

6. In the treatment of essential hypertension, beta-blockers are sufficient in the following racial groups:

A. Caucasians
B. Africans
C. Asians
D. Caribbeans
E. Chinese

7. Pernicious anaemia is rare among:

A. Europeans
B. Africans
C. Americans
D. Asians
E. Australians

8. A less severe variety of G6PD deficiency occurs:

A. in some 10% of African males
B. less frequently in European females
C. in some 10% of Irish males
D. less frequently in African females than African males
E. in some 10% of Asian males

9. **English height and weight charts do not apply to:**

A.   Afghans
B.   Bangladeshis
C.   Sri-Lankans
D.   Gujaratis
E.   South Indians

10. **Which of the following statements are true:**

A.   Abnormal haemoglobin C is common in West Africans
B.   Abnormal haemoglobin D is common in Punjabis
C.   Abnormal haemoglobin E is common in South-East Asians
D.   Beta thalassaemia is common in Cypriots
E.   Sickle-cell disease is common in Africans

CORRECT ANSWERS

1. B

2. C

3. D, C, B, E, A

4. A, B, D, E

5. C, E

6. A, C, E

7. B, D

8. A, D

9. B, C, D, E

10. A, B, C, D, E

ACKNOWLEDGEMENTS

I am grateful to the following organizations for giving permission to reprint various articles, as follows:

The Royal Society of Health:
Qureshi, B.A. (1981). Nutrition and multi-ethnic groups, *J. Roy. Soc. Health*, **101**, No. 5, Oct., pp.187–195
Qureshi, B.A. (1985). Family planning and culture. *J. Roy. Soc. Health*, **105**, No. 1, Feb., pp.11–14
Qureshi, B.A. (1985). Disease patterns in multi-ethnic groups in the UK. *J. Roy. Soc. Health*, **104**, No. 4, Oct., pp.153–155
Qureshi, B.A. (1986). Contraceptive advice: how the English differ from the Americans. *J. Roy. Soc. Health*, **106**(3), June, pp.77–79
Qureshi, B.A. (1986). Hidden corners of ethnic medical history. *J. Roy. Soc. Health*, **106**, No.5, October, pp.185–187

Modern Medicine:
Qureshi, B.A. (1982). Skin problems in ethnic Asians: avoiding diagnostic traps. *Modern Medicine*, **27**, No. 3, March, pp.28–29
Qureshi, B.A. (1984). Transcultural medicine. *Modern Medicine Promptcard*, Sept.

Rural Pharmacist:
Qureshi, B.A. (1982). Dangers of multi-therapy. *Rural Pharmacist*, No. 7, Nov., pp.9–10

Current Practice:
Qureshi, B.A. (1983). You offer but they need – gaps in the NHS care of multi-ethnic groups. *Current Practice*, No. 4, Feb., p.26

Newbourne Publications:
Qureshi, B.A. (1983). Understanding cultural customs and dangers of multi-therapy. *Primary Health Care*, **1**, No. 4, March, pp.9–10
Qureshi, B.A. (1986). Dealing with patients from different cultures. *Midwife, Health Visitor and Community Nurse*, **22**(12), December, pp.436–438 and 447

Royal College of General Practitioners:
Qureshi, B.A. (1983). The gap in the care of multi-ethnic groups, Report, RCGP 1983 Spring Meeting, Oxford, pp.29–30 (published by Thames Valley Faculty)
Qureshi, B.A. (1983–85). MRCGP Study Day for Overseas Graduates. *J. Roy. Coll. Gen. Practit.*, **33**, No. 251, June 83, p.381–2; **34**, No. 262, May 84, p. 290; **35**, No. 275, June 85, p.306
Qureshi, B.A, (1983–85). Annual Study Day for Overseas Graduates, *1983 RCGP Members' Reference Book*, p.100; *1984 RCGP Members' Reference Book*, p.119
Qureshi, B.A. (1983). Skin problems in multi-ethnic groups. *1983 RCGP Members' Reference Book*, pp.389–393
Qureshi, B.A. (1986). Nutritional problems in ethnic groups. *1986 RCGP Members' Reference Book*, pp.269–275

Pulse (Morgan Grampian Professional Press Ltd):

Qureshi, B.A. (1983). Patient care, cricket and transcultural confusion. *Pulse*, **48**(31), July 30, p.36

Qureshi, B.A. (1983). Transcultural medicine. *Pulse Reference Series*, **43**, Oct.29, pp.26–35; Nov.5 pp.35–44; Nov.12 pp.41–47

Qureshi, B.A. (1984). Beware when diagnosing 'battered Muslim children'. *Pulse*, **44**, Oct. 27, No. 42, p.43

Qureshi, B.A. (1985). Cultural conflicts in marriage and contraception. *Pulse Reference Series*, **45**, Jan. 26, pp.27–33

John Wright (Institute of Physics):

Qureshi, B.A. (1984). Muslim patients and the British GP. *The Medical Annual*, 1984, pp.259–271 (Bristol: John Wright)

Qureshi, B.A. (1986). Management of ethnic Asian patients in general practice. *The Medical Annual 1986*, ed. D.J. Pereira Gray, pp.155–65 (Bristol: John Wright)

Medical Publications Ltd:

Qureshi, B.A. (1984). Have a mind for Muslim matters. *GP*, June 29, p.21

Qureshi, B.A. (1984). Ethnic customs can affect the skin. *GP*, Sept. 28, p.33

Qureshi, B.A. (1985). Cultural needs in birth control. *GP*, April 5, p.33

British Medical Journal:

Qureshi, B.A. (1985). Multicultural Medicine series. *Br. Med.J.*, **290**, pp.1632, 1956; **291**, pp.790, 872, 1020; **294**, p.160; **295**, pp.818, 890

Qureshi, B.A. (1987). As she is spoke: Medicine and Books – Book review of 'English in Medicine'. *Br. Med. J.*, **294**, p.1607

Maternal and Child Health/Barker Publications Ltd:

Qureshi, B.A. (1985). Obstetric problems in multi-ethnic women. *Maternal and Child Health*, **10**(10), Oct., pp.303–307

Qureshi, B.A. (1987). Paediatric problems in multi-ethnic groups. *Maternal and Child Health*, **12**(1), Jan., pp.15–20

Cambridge University Press:

Qureshi, B.A., Farrah Sheikh, Donaldson, D., Morgan J.B. and Dickerson, J.W.T (1986). Birth weight and feeding practices of infants in Southall, Middx. *Proceedings of Nutritional Society*, **45**(2), p.60A

Family Planning Information Service:

Qureshi, B.A. (1986). Transcultural family planning consultations. *Family Planning Today*, (FPA & HEC), First quarter 1986, p.5

The Medical Tribune Group:

Qureshi, B.A. (1986). Skin problems encountered in multi-ethnic groups. *Dermatology in Practice*, **4**(4), August, pp.11–16

Prism International:

Qureshi, B.A. (1986). Skin diseases can pose problems for minorities. *Skin Concern*, p.6

Update-Siebert Publications Ltd:

Qureshi, B.A. (1988). Multicultural aspects of contraception. *Update: the Journal of Postgraduate General Practice*, **37**(5), Sept. 1, pp.406–410

I take this opportunity to thank the many colleagues who encouraged me in various stages of my research, especially Professor John Dickerson (Nutritionist), Drs David Donaldson (Consultant Pathologist), John Fry (GP and author), Howard Griffith (Editor of *Pulse*, Stephen Lock (Editor of *BMJ*), Dermot Lynch (GP and politician), Lotte Newman (Vice-Chairman of RCGP Council), Joyce Parker (Pharmacist), Denis Pereira-Gray (Chairman of RCGP Council), Jill Pereira-Gray (Assistant Editor RCGP Publications), Patrick Kerrigan (Medical Editor of *Pulse*), Richard Smith (Assistant Editor of *BMJ*), Keith Thompson (Examiner, MRCGP and DGM) and Freddie West (Editor of *Journal of the Royal Society of Health*).

I also thank Dr Peter Clarke (Publishing Director of Kluwer Academic Publishers, Medical Division) for his dedicated time, support and advice at all stages of preparation of this book. Phil Johnstone and Linda Thomas (Kluwer Academic Publishers) were most helpful in the final stages of production.

Finally, I extend my thanks to Jacqueline Priestley for her unfailing help and encouragement, and for typing the manuscripts and proof reading. Without her help this book would not have been written.

London, 1989   **BASHIR QURESHI**

INDEX